Alexandra König

The integration of new nursing staff from abroad

Alexandra König

The integration of new nursing staff from abroad

Challenges and burdens for existing nursing staff

ScienciaScripts

Imprint

Cover image: www.ingimage.com

This book is a translation from the original published under ISBN 978-620-0-44953-5.

Publisher:
Sciencia Scripts
is a trademark of
Dodo Books Indian Ocean Ltd. and OmniScriptum S.R.L publishing group

120 High Road, East Finchley, London, N2 9ED, United Kingdom
Str. Armeneasca 28/1, office 1, Chisinau MD-2012, Republic of Moldova, Europe
Printed at: see last page
ISBN: 978-620-8-28258-5

Contents

1 Summary

There has been a shortage of carers in the Austrian healthcare system for many years. Due to demographic developments, the picture for the future is alarming. The update of the nursing staff requirement forecast by Gesundheit Osterreich GmbH predicts an additional requirement of around 200,000 nursing staff by 2050. In order to maintain nursing operations, many operators of nursing facilities are pursuing the solution of integrating foreign nursing staff. This also applies to the company where I work as a care service manager, with 30 long-term care facilities in Austria. The integration of immigrant carers brings a lot of challenges in everyday life. Above all, the existing care teams in the individual care facilities are confronted with a range of additional tasks to familiarise themselves with the new colleagues and integrate them into society. The aim of this study was to shed light on the perspective of existing carers and to answer the questions of how they experience the integration process, which challenges and resources they describe and which support services they expect from management or which they consider to be helpful. For this purpose, a qualitative cross-sectional study and a case design were used by conducting 7 semi-structured interviews with existing carers from the group of companies, with and without a migration background. The statements from the interviews were then subjected to a qualitative content analysis and generalised. The results show that the existing carers experience stress due to the integration of foreign carers. Particularly in the areas of communication, which cannot be reduced to language skills, familiarisation, understanding of care and cultural differences, carers report challenging situations. The cause of this is primarily attributed to a lack of information, which is the responsibility of management. Many aspects of the challenges encountered are described in the literature and concepts and methods for the successful integration of foreign carers are cited. Little consideration is given to the perspective of existing carers. To improve the integration process, it is necessary to implement a well thought-out integration concept and to prepare both existing and foreign carers well. Management must be prepared to invest in financial and time resources in order to ensure the sustainable and successful integration of new immigrant carers.

For many years, there has been a shortage of health-care professionals in the Austrian healthcare system. Due to demographic trends, an alarming picture is emerging for the future. The update of the nursing staff demand forecast by 'Gesundheit Osterreich GmbH' predicts an additional need for around 200,000 caregivers by the year 2050. Many operators of care facilities pursue the approach of integrating foreign nursing professionals in order to maintain care operations. This is also the case for the Company i work for as a nursing manager, with 30 long-term care facilities in Austria. The integration of migrant health-care professionals brings a lot of challenges in everyday life. Especially the existing nursing teams in the individual care facilities are faced with a range of additional tasks for training and socially integrating new colleagues. The present study aimed to illuminate the perspective of existing health-care professionals and answer questions such as how they experience the integration process, what challenges and resources they describe, and what support they expect from management or find helpful from their point of view. A qualitative cross-sectional study and case design were applied, conducting 7 semi-structured interviews with existing health-care professionals from the Company, with and without migration background. The statements from the interviews were then subjected to qualitative content analysis and generalised. The results show that existing health-care professionals experience burdens from the integration of foreign carers. Particularly in the areas of communication, which cannot be reduced to language skills alone, training, understanding of care, and cultural differences, health-care professionals report challenging situations. The cause is mainly attributed to a lack of information, which is the responsibility of management. The literature describes many aspects of the expressed challenges in the present study and outlines concepts and methods for successful integration of foreign carers. The perspective of the existing professionals is given little consideration. To improve the integration process, it is necessary to implement a well-thought-out integration concept and prepare both existing and foreign healthcare professionals well. Management must be willing to invest financial and time resources to ensure sustainable and successful integration of new immigrant carers.

2 Definition of terms

COVID-19 pandemic

In December 2019, a novel coronavirus emerged in China that spread rapidly around the world and claimed around 6.5 million lives by the end of 2022. (Janssens et al., 2022)

Deductive/deduction

The term deduction means to derive or continue and describes the process of deriving knowledge from theory, it leads from the general to the particular. (Feustel, 2021)

Demography

The term demography describes population science, which focuses on the interrelationships of population processes with regard to economic, societal and social development. (Rohleder, 2012)

Discrimination

Discrimination is defined as behaviour or actions that intentionally belittle or disadvantage certain social groups or individuals belonging to these groups. (Hormel & Scherr, 2010)

Health professional register

The healthcare professions register serves to ensure quality assurance and patient safety and guarantees the traceability of who is authorised to practise the profession of healthcare and nursing as well as medical-technical services in the Austrian healthcare system. The Healthcare Register Professions Act was passed on 27 September 2016 for this purpose. Since 1 July 2018, the exercise of these professions has been subject to registration in the Health Professions Register. (Ministry of Social Affairs, 2024a)

Inductive/induction

The term induction means to bring about or cause and describes the process of developing a general validity of observations with the help of abstraction and generalisation of a theory. It leads from the particular to the general. (Feustel, 2021)

Intercultural

The dynamic process of exchange/interaction between different cultures is described as intercultural. (Bonacker & Geiger, 2021)

Migration

Migration is derived from the Latin word *migrare*, which means to wander or move away. This general definition does not take into account temporal, spatial or personal factors. In the past, the term "wandering" or "migratory movement" was used. The word *migration* has its origins in publications from the 1930s. Today, migration is defined in a political and legal context and described as a change of residence or crossing borders, whereby the reason for migration is not differentiated. (Hahn, 2023)

Multicultural

Multicultural is described as the state of many cultures existing side by side without interacting with each other. (Bonacker & Geiger, 2021)

Nostrification procedure

Nostrification is a procedure for recognising a school or university degree obtained abroad for the purpose of practising a profession. (Ministry of Social Affairs, 2024b)

Pseudonymise

The pseudonymisation of data in the research process aims to limit the assignment of individual data sets to specific persons or to make it controllable. (Dewes, 2022)

Stereotyping

Stereotyping is the attribution of certain characteristics to a group of people. Typical characteristics and behaviours are associated with this group. (Winter & Sassenberg, 2022)

Transcribing/transcription

The process of writing down the spoken word from interviews or videos in qualitative data analysis is called transcription. It forms the basis for analysing the data. (Mayer, 2022)

Validity

Validity in research makes it possible to assess the study design and is categorised into internal and external validity.

Internal validity makes it possible to conclude that the dependent variable is influenced by the independent variable. This means that the internal validity informs whether other possibilities are possible for a change in the dependent variable than the influence of the independent variable.

External validity provides information about the relevance of the study and for whom or in which setting the results of the research can be generalised. (Mayer, 2022)

3 Introduction

The aim of this work is to take a closer look at the perspective of existing nursing staff on the integration of nursing staff who have immigrated from abroad and to present their experiences in order to be able to draw practical benefits from them.
The shortage of skilled nursing staff is well known, but has become even more dramatic as a result of the COVID-19 pandemic. The result is blocked beds in acute inpatient and outpatient settings, as well as a decline in the quality of care for patients. There are many measures and solutions. One of these is the acquisition of nursing staff from abroad. The process of integrating foreign carers poses a number of challenges for institutions, management and teams. Many of these have already been considered and are described in the literature. The problems that nursing staff of foreign origin have to overcome have already been analysed in a number of studies. The main problem areas are the language barrier, the culture, cases of discrimination and the different training system in the country of origin. These issues are covered in detail in the literature, as is the complicated and time-consuming process of having professional qualifications acquired abroad recognised. The situation of managers and the challenges they face in dealing with foreign carers is well illustrated in the literature. The endeavours of politicians and healthcare institutions to keep nurses who have immigrated from abroad in Austria and in the profession are clearly evident. In practice, the familiarisation and integration of foreign nursing staff creates burdens for existing nursing staff in particular, but also positive developments that have not yet been included in the considerations and research.
The answers to the research questions will clarify which measures and steps are necessary to accelerate the process of integrating care workers who have migrated from abroad and to improve the quality of cooperation.
The results were obtained using semi-structured interviews with nursing staff from the company in which the author works as a nursing manager. The participants for the interviews were recruited from a total of around 800 nursing staff. This means that the results are also very meaningful.
In the literature section, the shortage of skilled labour and the use of foreign nursing staff was described as a solution. Integration and the problem areas that can arise in the process were also described.
The empirical part is divided into the method, results and discussion sections. The methods section presents the aim of the work and the research questions, as well as the interview method according to Witzel and the results analysis according to Mayring. The recruitment of participants, field access and research ethics are also described in the methods section. The data obtained from the interviews is visualised in the results section. In the discussion, the results are compared with the descriptions in the literature.

1.1 Demographic trends and the shortage of skilled nursing staff

There has been a shortage of nursing staff in Austria for many years. One of the main reasons is certainly the demographic development. Due to improved living conditions, life expectancy is continuously increasing. (Bettig et al., 2012) The population structure is characterised by low birth rates and high life expectancy. Despite this, the total population in Austria has been rising steadily for decades, which is due not only to the development of increasing life expectancy but also to immigration from abroad. (Fent et al., 2019)

According to the 2019 nursing staff requirement forecast by Gesundheit Osterreich GmbH (GOG), Austria's total population will grow by around 6 per cent by 2030. Of this, 25 per cent will be accounted for by people aged 75 and over. The number of people aged between 85 and 89 is even forecast to grow by 50 per cent. Consequently, the need for care and the complexity of care settings increase with age. (Rappold & Juraszovich, 2019)

At the same time, the need for highly qualified nursing staff is increasing and, in light of the COVID-19 pandemic, which has exacerbated the shortage of nursing staff, a difficult future scenario is emerging. (Tahic, 2023)

It is becoming increasingly difficult for the providers of care facilities to ensure an adequate number and quality of nursing staff to care for the patients. There are massive shortages in day-to-day care and this is exacerbated by the fact that many carers will be retiring in the near future. In 2019, 1/3 of carers were already aged 50 or older, according to the Healthcare Professionals Register. Conversely, the number of young people entering the healthcare and nursing profession is falling. (Rappold & Juraszovich, 2019)

In order to increase the attractiveness and professionalisation of the training of senior healthcare and nursing staff, it was raised to the tertiary level and the professional groups were redefined with the 2016 amendment to the GuKG. Despite these changes, the number of nursing graduates has stagnated. The number of people starting nursing training is even declining. (Pleschberger & Holzweber, 2019)

As a result, the shortage occupation list, which has been published in the Federal Ministry of Labour's Skilled Workers Ordinance since 2012, has also included healthcare and nursing since 2021. All three occupational groups of the Healthcare and Nursing Act - *qualified nurses, nursing assistants and care assistants* - are listed. (Gleitsmann et al., 2022)

There is also a high proportion of part-time employees in the care sector. In the area of long-term care, 13 nursing professionals were already needed to fill 10 full-time positions in 2017. (Rappold & Juraszovich, 2019)

Another key influencing factor is the high workload in the care sector. Both physical and mental stress lead to early departures from the nursing profession before retirement. The working climate index of the Federal Ministry of Social Affairs, Health, Care and Consumer Protection on working conditions in the nursing professions from 2021 - in which 4,000 employees from the healthcare and nursing sector were surveyed - showed high percentage points in nursing and geriatric care, especially in the areas of *time pressure* and *mentally stressful work*, as shown in Figure 1. (Schonherr, 2021)

Loads	**Nursing care**	**Elderly care**	**Care for the**	**Other**

			disabled	Professions
Time pressure	32%	32%	14%	22%
Mentally stressful work	46%	38%	41%	11%
Change of work processes	18%	18%	14%	10%
constant work pressure without time to catch your breath	24%	23%	10%	15%
Accident and Risk of injury	14%	10%	11%	11%

Figure 1: Subjective workload in the care professions. Employees who stated that they felt "very" or "fairly" stressed in the individual areas. Source: Austrian Work Climate Index, 2021.

There are a number of ideas on how to tackle the shortage of skilled nursing staff. One solution is the integration of foreign nursing staff. The possibilities of integrating skilled nursing staff and the challenges and opportunities that arise from this will be discussed in more detail in the next chapter.

1.2 The deployment of foreign carers as a solution

The shortage of nursing staff described in Chapter 3.1 requires a series of measures to ensure the continued care of patients and residents in long-term care facilities. Those responsible in politics and business have recognised that the recruitment of nursing staff from abroad is a key component in solving the problem. (Bossle & Kunhardt, 2022) However, the migration of carers to Austria is not a new phenomenon. The city of Vienna recruited Serbian qualified nurses as early as 1967 and the proud number of 700 Filipino nurses in 1974. (Lenhart, 2018)

3.2.1 Reasons for migration in the care sector in Austria

With a total population of around 8.8 million people in 2020, 24.4 per cent already had a migrant background. The reasons for recruiting nurses from abroad are clear due to the staff shortage. The reasons for nurses to emigrate to Austria are mainly due to the conditions in their countries of origin. (Bachinger, 2009)

There are so-called *"push and pull factors"* that motivate nurses of foreign origin to leave their country. Pull factors are

These are the motivating factors that motivate carers to emigrate to an attractive destination country. Push factors, on the other hand, are negatively triggered and arise from conditions in their own country that cause them to leave their country of origin. (Kline, 2003)

Table 1 Push and pull factors. (Kline, 2003)

Push factors	**Pull factors**	**Category**
No professional development	Good professional	Education/Career
Limited exercise of nursing	development opportunities	Education/Career
skills	Training in nursing skills	Economic efficiency
Poor pay, low standard of living	possible Good pay, high standard of living	Political/Social

High personal risk	High personal security

The topic of migration is more important than ever for the care sector today. Worldwide crises, social and political developments and globalisation are causing nurses to emigrate to economically strong countries. On the other hand, it is essential for Austria and the prevailing conditions of massive staff shortages to recruit nurses from abroad. (Goldgruber et al., 2023)

Recruitment service providers and placement agencies play a decisive role here. For employers, hiring recruitment agencies for the recruitment of foreign nurses is a huge relief because the agencies usually take care of all the necessary steps for entry and subsequently for the start of work. Nevertheless, recruitment agencies should be viewed critically, as they know what qualities an employee should have in order to be attractive to potential employers. In this way, the perception and image of employers is specifically shaped by the agencies. (Bossle & Kunhardt, 2022)

According to the GOG's annual report on the register of healthcare professionals, the proportion of nurses from all professional groups (DGKP, PFA, PA) who completed their training abroad was 11 per cent. (Holzweber et al., 2022)

In order to recruit nurses from abroad and employ them in Austria, there are a number of official requirements that need to be met. The topic of professional recognition is therefore dealt with in the next chapter.

3.2.2 Nostrification procedures and the recognition of foreign professional qualifications in nursing

In order for nurses from abroad to be able to work professionally in Austria, it is necessary to have their professional qualification recognised. The procedure for this is enshrined in law in the European Directive on the Recognition of Professional Qualifications (2005/36/EC). As the training systems in the various countries differ, it is also necessary to check the content of the professional qualification. This serves to ensure the safety of carers in the acute and extramural care sector. The recognition procedure applies to nurses from EU member states, EEA signatory states or the Swiss Confederation. All other nursing professionals who come from so-called third countries must undergo a nostrification procedure. (Bachinger, 2009)

3.2.2.1 The recognition procedure

In order for the professional qualification to be recognised, nurses must provide proof of successful completion of their nursing training in the form of a certificate (diploma, certificate, etc.). Recognition of the professional qualification is also possible for nurses from third countries, provided they already have a professional licence in an EU state, an EEA contracting state or the Swiss Confederation and have proof that they have worked in the recognised profession in this state for at least 3 years. In addition to the personal documents, the applicant nurses must provide an officially certified document confirming that the professional qualification acquired abroad complies with the Professional Qualifications Directive 2005/36/EC. Furthermore, confirmation from the country of origin is required that the exercise of the profession has not been temporarily or definitively prohibited. (Ministry of Social Affairs, 2023)

Care assistant professions are also obliged to enclose a curriculum and certificates of employment. All documents to be submitted must be originals and require a notarised translation into German. The application for recognition of the professional qualification is made directly to the Federal Ministry of Social Affairs, Health and Consumer Protection. (Ministry of Social Affairs, 2023)

3.2.2.2 The nostrification procedure

As already mentioned, the equivalence of training in the country of origin is checked for nurses from a third country in the so-called nostrification procedure. The condition applies to qualified healthcare and nursing staff.

Nurses must apply to the universities of applied sciences that offer a relevant degree programme. For the nursing assistant professions, however, applications must be submitted to the respective provincial governor. (Ministry of Social Affairs, 2023)

3.2.2.3 The red-white-red card

The "Red-White-Red Card", which was introduced in 2011 as part of the Aliens Law Amendment Act, facilitates access to the Austrian labour market. This makes it easier for skilled workers from shortage occupations to work in Austria if they already have a job. This makes it possible for third-country nationals to take up employment even before the nostrification procedure has been completed. (Krings, 2013)

1.3 Problem areas in the integration of foreign carers into the care service

Care teams with employees from different backgrounds are often found in everyday care work. The heterogeneity in these groups creates a number of challenges that need to be overcome, but also opportunities that need to be utilised. The problem of understanding and language barriers is obvious, but there are other factors that need to be taken into account. Different cultures, values and ways of communicating should also be considered. (Bossle & Kunhardt, 2022)

Discrimination is a particularly sensitive issue. The study *"Experiences of discrimination in Germany"* showed that 26.4 per cent of nursing staff have been confronted with discriminatory behaviour. Often in the context of racially motivated backgrounds. (Stolle-Wahl & Reinhardt, 2022)

This chapter deals with the most important problem areas that can arise from the integration of foreign nursing professionals.

3.3.1 Communication and language barriers

The linguistic conflict between caregivers with different mother tongues is one of the biggest hurdles in everyday care work and is exacerbated by the different dialects in the countries. (Goldgruber et al., 2023)

Passing on information in dialect can lead to misunderstandings among carers from abroad and subsequently trigger conflicts within the team. In contrast, speaking in High German has a positive effect on understanding. (Bossle & Kunhardt, 2022)

Dialect language among the team members that nurses of other native languages cannot follow leads to insecurity and marginalisation. Fear and a feeling of social exclusion can arise for the carer who does not understand the conversation. Emerging thoughts that the content of the conversation could be about them lead to illness or anger. A language consists of more than just words and grammar. Linguistic and cultural characteristics also have an effect on communication, as do vocabulary and sentence structure. The meaning of words and the content of information must be paraphrased and explained so that carers with a different mother tongue can understand what is being said. Communication within the care team is one of the most important building blocks for ensuring nursing quality. Care measures are planned and carried out on the basis of an understanding of the spoken information, its content and meaning. Every carer in the team must be able to pass on important nursing information orally and in writing. (Ertl et al., 2022)

Working with nursing documentation is a particular challenge for foreign nursing staff. Writing down nursing events and information becomes more difficult if the appropriate vocabulary has not yet been developed. This problem is exacerbated by the prevailing time pressure in everyday nursing care. The interlinked thinking of nursing knowledge and language is particularly evident in the writing of technical content, such as the preparation of the nursing report. The creation of care plans in everyday life is suitable for practising this. Common expressions used in the various care situations should be explained to the foreign carers. Through constant repetition, these phrases and terms can subsequently be recalled and understood by all care professionals. (Bossle & Kunhardt, 2022)

Written documentation is particularly important in order to avoid loss of information and to ensure that the day-to-day running of a long-term care facility runs smoothly. The care report has a special role to play here. Nursing staff who have immigrated from abroad are under pressure because, in practice, incorrect spelling or grammar often leads to criticism from domestic colleagues. This sometimes results in an attempt to avoid these errors by asking existing colleagues to take over for them. Another strategy is the use of standardised phrases, which means that the written information is incomplete and not very meaningful in terms of content. In addition, there are requirements to include only essential information in the care report and to keep it brief. As this is also a challenge for Austrian carers, it is an even greater challenge for carers of foreign origin.

Hurde. A clear guideline for creating written care documentation can be of great benefit to an intercultural team. A respectful approach and an open error culture in the context of documentation reduce tensions and misunderstandings in the team. (Ertl et al., 2022)

3.3.2 Cultural differences

In contrast to medicine, nursing care in Europe is a profession shaped by history and culture. The accompaniment and support of elderly people in the activities of daily life - eating and drinking, movement, elimination, washing and dressing,

communication, safety - which are the centre of nursing activities in the Austrian nursing culture, are often perceived as inferior activities by nursing professionals from abroad. In many countries, these services are provided by relatives and care there is strongly characterised by medical activities. (Zegelin, 2023)
In order to utilise the resources that a team of carers from several different cultures has, it is necessary to achieve cultural openness. Without an intercultural orientation of the company, prejudices against a culture are reinforced, which are projected onto the individual foreign carers who belong to this culture. Immigrant nurses are thus exposed to stereotyping based on the prejudices of their culture. (Bachinger, 2009)
However, employers also attribute certain qualities to foreign nursing professionals. They are considered highly qualified due to their tertiary-level training. As the earning potential in Austria is usually much higher than in their country of origin, employers also believe that migrant nurses are more motivated and more willing to work overtime. The attributed characteristics can therefore have both positive and negative effects. Conflict situations on a professional or organisational level that are shifted to the cultural level are problematic. The reason for this lies in an excessive focus on the foreign culture on an operational basis. The actual origin of the conflict is not recognised. (Bossle, 2022)
Multicultural care teams tend to exclude heterogeneity in the team and ascribe identical role models and behaviours to all members. However, this also leads to the exclusion of different resources, as a result of which foreign nursing staff feel burdened and discriminated against because specific skills that they bring with them cannot be utilised. It is therefore not only important to counteract prejudices, but also to build up tolerance for other experiences and skills. (Bachinger, 2009)

3.3.3 The management

Leadership in the care sector has also changed in recent years and decades due to demographic and structural developments. The personnel management of a multicultural team is a particular challenge. Ward and department managers have a special role to play here in direct contact with the nursing staff. Managers face major hurdles when familiarising themselves with new foreign colleagues due to a lack of language skills. They have to be very flexible and deviate from established guidelines if necessary. When assigning foreign nursing staff for induction, ward and department managers are increasingly criticised by the existing nursing staff in the team, as they are also overwhelmed by the situation. Leading and managing multicultural teams requires intercultural competence in dealing with the different attitudes towards care and dealing with health and illness. It is not enough to structure and organise everyday nursing care. Different behaviours in dealing with pain, dying or fear require reinterpretation within the team as a whole. (Angelovski, 2014)
This means that the leadership must guide the team members in their behaviour so that a uniform approach is achieved in certain settings. Two leadership styles are decisive for the management of a team. Task-orientated leadership, which serves to achieve goals, and employee-orientated leadership, which serves to

maintain the team with its social component. Now it seems simple if the ward or area manager of a multicultural team focusses on task-oriented leadership, thus relieving the team of the responsibility for shaping its own processes and making everyday care easier by reducing the potential for conflict. Conflicts nevertheless occur in every team and, as there is also a specific norm for dealing with and resolving conflicts in task-oriented management, it can be assumed that the different behavioural patterns in multicultural teams will lead to an intensification of the respective conflict. It should also be borne in mind that motivation decreases when nursing staff are no longer able to contribute to the organisation of their workplace and their expertise is no longer taken into account. This is why employee-orientated leadership is essential for multicultural teams. A manager who demonstrates openness in communication and towards different cultures can influence different behaviours and attitudes and manage team processes better. (Bachmann & Wolf, 2007)

As teaching intercultural and multicultural skills to care managers is a key factor for the successful integration of new care workers from abroad, operators of long-term care facilities are particularly challenged. Basic and intermediate care managers should be prepared for the new challenges in further and advanced training programmes. (Angelovski, 2014)

3.3.4 Training systems in the countries of origin of migrant nurses

According to the factsheet on facts and figures from the health professions register from 2022, a total of 11 per cent of registered nurses in Austria acquired their professional qualification abroad. 3 per cent of them in a third country. (Holzweber et al., 2022)

In the Austrian healthcare and nursing curriculum, so-called basic care - i.e. the orientation of nursing measures towards the "activities of daily living" - forms the basis for all nursing activities. (Rottenhofer et al., 2003)

This includes compensatory support for deficits such as washing, dressing or defecating. In many countries - including the Philippines, Bosnia, Serbia and India - these activities are carried out by relatives and are not seen as a care task. As a result, these care activities are not part of the training. (Herlach, 2021)

Since many of the nurses who have immigrated from abroad come to us from the Balkan region and Filipino nurses have been emigrating to Austria to work in the nursing profession for decades, the training systems of these two countries were used as examples in this study.

Nursing training in the Philippines can be completed both at universities and at private nursing schools and culminates in a Bachelor of Sciences in Nursing. In addition to the nursing and medical subject area, general education subjects such as maths and English are also part of the curriculum. With 2106 hours of theoretical and 1578 hours of practical training, the total number of hours and above all the practical hours is lower than in Austria, where a total of 4600 hours - including 2300 hours of practical training - is stipulated by law. During their studies, nursing students have the opportunity to specialise in one area (hospital nursing, community nursing, palliative care, school nursing, psychiatric nursing, geriatric nursing, clinical nursing). Although basic care is not included in the training, a 6-month course called *Caregiving II* is offered, which teaches the skills of basic care. (Fulda University of Applied Sciences, 2020b)

In Bosnia and Herzegovina, nursing training is offered after compulsory schooling at secondary medical schools, which are known as *middle-level medical schools*. General education subjects are also taught during the four-year training programme, which means that the number of hours of theory and 990 hours of practical training specific to the nursing profession is significantly lower than in Austria at 891 hours. An internship is only completed after the training programme and lasts just 6 months. There is then the option of studying for a Bachelor's degree at various universities. As there is no difference in the level of responsibility between graduates *of middle-level medical schools* and academically trained nurses in everyday working life, only 1 per cent of Bosnian nurses have a bachelor's degree. Basic nursing care is also not included in the training content in Bosnia and Herzegovina. As in the Philippines, this is provided by the relatives of the carers. (HochschuleFulda, 2020a) Nurses from these countries who emigrate to Austria to practise the nursing profession here are initially confronted with the unfamiliar task of basic care. This results in problems with the basic understanding of care between nurses who have completed their training in Austria and the immigrant nurses.

1.4 The research gap

The results from the empirical data described in the literature primarily highlight challenges from the perspective of the migrant carers. In addition, problems that can arise in cooperation and in the team are presented. Solution strategies and experiences from pilot projects aimed at improving integration are also taken into account. Although the existing nursing staff play an essential role in familiarisation and social integration into the team, there is very limited empirical data on their experiences. Due to the increased acquisition of foreign nursing staff, there is a need for studies on what support existing nursing staff require during familiarisation and integration. Surveying the views of existing nursing staff and their experiences in the context of communication, the culturally determined different behaviours and attitudes can be a resource for the development of a new culture.

improvement of the integration process. The data collected was used to analyse challenges, misunderstandings and barriers and subsequently develop strategies to counter them. Closing the research gap should help to improve the quality of the integration process, also with regard to resident care. A typical case was used to research the topic for this thesis.

4 Research question and objective

This work attempts to present the perspective of existing nursing staff, their experiences and their experiences of the integration of nursing staff who have immigrated from abroad into the nursing service.

This gives rise to the following research questions:

- How do existing nursing staff experience the integration of new nursing staff from abroad into long-term care facilities?
- What challenges and resources does the existing nursing staff describe during familiarisation and integration?
- What support services can be provided by managers from the perspective of existing carers and what measures are necessary to improve the quality of cooperation and accelerate the integration process?

The results of the data collection should be used to generate targeted measures that simplify the familiarisation of foreign nursing staff for existing nursing staff and subsequently improve the quality of resident care. The research objective of the thesis is to generate targeted measures for improving the integration process and increasing the quality of cooperation between the teams by utilising the solutions and resources from the perspective of existing nursing staff.

1.1 Research design and method

As the subjective perspective of existing carers and their experience of the induction of new carers from abroad is the focus of this work, a qualitative approach was chosen. The qualitative research process is characterised by not limiting the research to one method, but remaining flexible by using a wide range of methods to achieve the research objective. It is essential that the choice of research method is adapted to the subject of the study. Qualitative research is orientated towards everyday events and people's everyday knowledge. The focus is on experiences and subjective reality, which is characterised by everyday life. The guiding principle of qualitative research is the consideration of statements and actions in the context of their environment and framework conditions, taking into account the perspectives of those involved. A basic prerequisite is the reflexivity of the researcher to be aware of his/her role in the research process and the fact that he/she is interacting with the object of research. Understanding is the epistemological principle of qualitative research in order to develop an understanding of subjective perspectives and social aspects. The willingness to accept new perspectives and information according to the principle of openness must be given for the researcher. The starting point is the case analysis, which makes it possible to develop a deeper understanding of a specific case or a limited number of cases and enables a construction of reality as a basis. This means that reality is not objective and is constructed by people through perception and interpretation. Qualitative research as textual science refers to the collection of data in text form. The analysis of this data, from interviews, written texts, discussions, etc., represents the centre of the research work and provides insight into people's subjective realities. Discovery and theorising are the clear aim of qualitative research in order to gain new insights that can serve as the basis for further research. (Flick et al., 2009)

1.2 Study design

A qualitative cross-sectional study and a case design were chosen for the study design. Mayer (2022) describes the "*bounded system*", i.e. a limited and closed system, as one of the main criteria for a qualitative case study. The study was carried out in a sponsoring organisation that provides long-term care and thus represents the *bounded system*. (Mayer, 2022) The organisation has 30 locations with around 800 employees. The shortage of skilled workers in care facilities is also an everyday occurrence in this company, and the acquisition of new care professionals is proving to be extremely difficult. For this reason, the management is recruiting nursing staff from abroad via various recruitment agencies. The main focus is on recruiting new employees from Slovenia and Croatia. In order to utilise even more channels for recruitment, the company has also started to recruit specialists from third countries such as Bosnia and Herzegovina, Tunisia, the Philippines and Colombia. When training the new recruits from

The arrival of nursing staff from abroad poses challenges that existing nursing staff describe as a particular burden. This burden is the phenomenon to be analysed in the study.

The qualitative case study serves not only to describe a phenomenon, but also to develop a deeper, holistic understanding in order to be able to verify or generate theories. To do this, the phenomenon must always be analysed in the context of all influencing factors, the lifeworld. (Mayer, 2022) This makes it possible to see things from different perspectives. For this reason, the interviews in this thesis were conducted with carers from different locations and occupational groups.

1.3 Field access, recruitment and sampling

As mentioned in Chapter 5.1, the research field was limited to the care facilities of one company in Austria. The field was accessed hierarchically via the management.

For the recruitment, an information letter describing the background and purpose of this work, as well as a consent form, was sent to the nursing home managers. They informed the nursing staff in their own organisation, who were able to contact the researcher on a voluntary basis. Open questions were clarified by telephone with the interested carers and the interview appointments were arranged. The study is limited to long-term care facilities and their nursing staff who provide basic nursing care and are confronted with the familiarisation and cooperation with new nursing staff from abroad in their everyday work. The sampling was therefore criteria-based and selective. The following inclusion and exclusion criteria were defined for the participants:

Table 2: Inclusion and exclusion criteria for participation in the study. (own presentation).

Inclusion criteria	Exclusion criteria
Qualified carers	Executives
Nursing assistants	Employees of personnel leasing companies

With and without a migration background	School pupils and students
Length of service 1 year or longer	Employees from the domestic care sector
At least 5 years of professional experience in healthcare and nursing in Eastern Europe	

For the study, it seemed particularly interesting to also collect the views of existing carers with a migration background, who were themselves in the role of newly arrived carers and therefore know both perspectives on the integration process. When drawing the sample, an attempt was made to recruit as broadly as possible in the sense of *theoretical sampling.* The participants were selected from different locations in order to include different perspectives. When selecting the interviewees, an attempt was made to recruit further interviewees based on the initial results of the interviews in order to gain new and further insights.

1.4 Method of data collection

Semi-structured, guideline-based, problem-centred individual interviews according to Witzel were conducted to collect the data.

The concept of problem-centredness describes a specific problem or phenomenon that is perceived and investigated by the researcher. This involves researching the background knowledge and then systematising it from the existing literature. Another essential part of the study is the collection and integration of the experts' experiences in the form of interviews. The interview guide, in which the topics of the study were systematically formulated in questions, serves to orientate the researcher. However, the focus of the interview is on the course of the conversation with the interviewed expert. This allows the researcher to ask specific follow-up questions that serve the cognitive interest of the research subject. (Witzel, 1985)

Based on the existing knowledge and the author's own expertise, as well as the research questions, an interview guide with a total of 21 questions and sub-questions was created for the interviews. A total of seven interviews were conducted in the period from January 2024 to February 2024. Six interviews could be conducted in person, one had to be conducted virtually via MS teams due to the great distance. Three of the participants are qualified nurses, four have the qualification of nursing assistant, two of whom have a migrant background themselves. The interviews were conducted in the care facilities where the interview partners work, in an undisturbed room provided by the respective care service management. The majority of the interviews lasted between 30 and 45 minutes.

1.5 Data management and data protection

The interviews were transcribed using a semantic-content transcription system. (Dresing & Pehl, 2015)

The data was then pseudonymised, i.e. names and other identifying features were replaced by codes and subsequently stored in a secure location to protect against unauthorised access. The declarations of consent were also stored in a separate, secure location.

1.6 Analysing the data

The transcribed and pseudonymised interviews and the resulting data were analysed using qualitative content analysis according to Mayring (2022). Content analysis is a reductive procedure on a manifest level in which the data is structured systematically and reduced to content-relevant statements. (Mayring, 2022)

For this purpose, deductive categories - which are based on the research questions and the findings from the literature - were formed according to the 7 phases of the structuring qualitative content analysis by Kukartz (2018). Inductive categories were supplemented in the course of the analysis process and data that had already been analysed underwent a second coding process. (Kuckartz, 2018)

The coding process was carried out with software support using the MAXQDA programme. Following Mayring's (2022) process model, the categorisation was followed by paraphrasing, generalisation and reduction of the data in order to be able to summarise it according to subject area. (Mayring, 2022)

1.7 Good criteria and validity justification

In order to ensure quality, validity and reliability in qualitative social research, research work based on good criteria is of great importance.

According to Mayring (2016), six method-specific good criteria are applied, on the basis of which the research results can be checked for their suitability. The importance of **procedural documentation** is described so that the research process is comprehensible for everyone. The steps of the research process are also documented in this work with the information letter, the declaration of consent, the recorded interviews and their transcription and the analysis protocols. **The interpretations** of the data resulting from the analysis are comprehensible and substantiated with the **argumentative interpretation validation**. The steps of the derived interpretation can be seen in the analysis protocols. Furthermore, the analyses and data were discussed with the supervisor of the thesis, Dr.

Simon Krutter, who is very experienced in qualitative research, was discussed. In order to ensure a systematic collection of data and a systematic processing of the data, it is essential that the procedure **is guided by rules** without, however, having to exclude openness towards the subject matter. All steps of the analysis procedure were carried out according to the methodology of qualitative content analysis according to Mayring (2022) and the data were analysed uniformly in accordance with this procedure. Since object-appropriateness is the guiding principle of qualitative research, **proximity to the object** is an essential component. The research takes place as close as possible to the lifeworld of those being researched - the field. The author's work as a care service manager in the company and the fact that the interviews were conducted in the professional context of the participants ensures proximity to the subject of the research. In order to strengthen the quality of the research, **triangulation** is used by carrying out several analyses. This also involves combining different data sources and applying several methods. The data from the various interviews was collated and analysed. Furthermore, data that had already been evaluated was subjected to further analyses after the formation of inductive categories that emerged during the categorisation. Finally, **communicative validation** was used to validate the research results. The results are presented to the interviewees and if they recognise themselves in them, this is an essential feature for validating the research results. The focus is not on complete agreement, but on assessing the strengths and weaknesses of the research work. The work is made available to the participants for viewing and the results for discussion. (Mayring, 2016)

1.8 Ethical reflection

As the study was a survey, participation was voluntary and the participants were not a vulnerable group of people, no ethics vote was observed. All aspects of ethics and data protection were discussed with the author's supervisor, Dr Simon Krutter. As already mentioned, access to the field was hierarchically via the management of the organisation, which granted permission to conduct the study. The approval of the works council and the head of the Human Resources department was also obtained. The participants learnt about the study from the nursing service management of the care facility in which they work. If they were interested, they were given the information letter and the consent form. The information letter explicitly emphasised the voluntary nature of participation, the data protection and the anonymisation of the data. The possibility of cancelling participation at any time is also mentioned in the information letter. Those interested were given the researcher's contact details in order to clarify any open questions and, if they had decided to participate, to arrange appointments for the interviews to be conducted. Before the interviews, all participants were once again informed about the procedure. Any remaining open questions were answered. All interested parties decided to participate. The consent forms were drawn up in duplicate and signed by both the participants and the researcher.

5 results

This chapter summarises the results of the interviews. As already mentioned, 7 interviews were conducted with carers from the company group. Two carers with a migrant background, who themselves joined the care service in Austria years ago, were also recruited for the survey.

Table 3 Sample description

Gender	1 male carer	6 female carers
Average age	41.14 years (28 to 63 years)	
Qualification	3 qualified carers	4 care assistants
Origin	5 from Austria	2 with a migration background
Professional experience	5 to 15 years	
Company affiliation	2 to 15 years	

In addition to the major challenges that arise in the integration process, many resources and positive changes were also perceived. The results are listed according to the categories from the analysis of the interviews. Some categories were formed deductively in advance and expanded to include inductive categories that emerged from the analysis process. The categories are first used to describe the general view of the interviewees on the solution approach of integrating international nursing staff for the shortage of skilled labour. This is followed by an assessment of the immigrant nurses' contrasting understanding of care in connection with training. In the next section, the professional areas of quality, assumption of responsibility and the

familiarisation process. In addition to technical aspects, social interaction and the subjective experience of the nursing staff interviewed are the most important part of the results. Here, communication and teamwork, social integration and culture are experienced as particularly challenging. The last part deals with leadership, how the experts experience it in the integration process and what expectations they have of the managers. It also looks at the resource-orientated approach of relieving the burden by integrating foreign carers.

Table 4: Main and sub-categories of the data analysis

Main categories	Subcategories
Integration as a solution	
	Preparation for the field of activity
Professional quality	
Assumption of responsibility	
Team	
	Empathy
	Co-operation
	Cohesion
	Extra work due to stress
Integration as a relief	
	Advantages through integration

Category	Subcategory
Familiarisation	
	Operational readiness
	Familiarisation period
	Willingness to learn
Social integration	
	Willingness to integrate
	Gender differences
Education	
	Care documentation
	Differences
Guidance	
Culture	
	Residents' reactions
	Dealing with residents
	Behaviour
Communication	
	Information for existing employees
	Language

5.1 The integration of foreign nursing staff as a solution to the shortage of skilled nursing staff

Many of the interview participants see the recruitment of foreign nursing staff to counteract the tense staffing situation in a positive light. However, this is not a general solution to the shortage of carers in Austria. The fact that immigrant nurses are employed at a rate of 100 per cent is seen as an advantage due to the increasing work pressure. However, all of the nursing staff surveyed criticised the inadequate preparation of the immigrant carers and the immature integration process. In particular, the preparation of foreign carers for the field of nursing in Austria, the lack of language skills and the different understanding of nursing were criticised. Two of the interviewees were rather critical of the deployment of foreign carers and saw shortcomings, especially in politics. One of the carers interviewed pointed out that the problem of the shortage of skilled workers has been known for decades and nothing has been done about it or it has even been deliberately controlled. The situation of immigrant carers was also criticised. Recruiting carers from abroad who have to leave their home country and leave their families behind for various reasons was described as exploitation.

"They are being exploited. They have to go abroad, as do the carers. I don't think it's funny when they have to go there for two months and leave the little children alone. They don't even ask core r...." (IB, segment3)

The nursing staff interviewed see solutions to the shortage of skilled workers in making the nursing profession more attractive with better pay, the expansion of outpatient care and more support for family carers.

5.2 The contrasting understanding of nursing care among foreign nursing professionals

The area of responsibility in the country of origin of foreign carers usually differs from that in Austria. In their qualification as qualified nurses, they mainly worked in the medical-therapeutic field. In everyday nursing care, the nurses interviewed perceive the high level of competence of the immigrant nurses in this area, but emphasised a lack of competence in basic care.

"I know they were probably graduates there, or I don't know. Maybe they weren't in nursing? But we're in nursing now, we're not there as graduates with medication and everything." (IA, segment 2)

In Austria, especially in long-term care, working in basic nursing care is an essential part of the job. In addition, there is the care concept of person-centred, holistic care, which is a new and unfamiliar approach for the immigrant nurses. The understanding of care differs greatly from that of the existing carers, who focus on the holistic care of the residents in their work. The experts describe conveying an understanding of the content of person-centred care as particularly difficult due to language deficits. The carers interviewed now know that in many countries, such as the Philippines or Tunisia, basic care is provided by the close relatives of the person being cared for. They therefore consider it particularly important to inform foreign carers about the field of care in Austria so that the migrant carers know what to expect. The nurses interviewed criticised the fact that they did not receive any information in advance about the training content and area of activity of their new foreign colleagues.

"And I also don't know how they run their elderly care. I have no idea if there's anything or anything else. Or I assume they are cared for in the family, like we were 30 or 40 years ago." (IB, Segment7)

They stated that they had assumed that immigrant nurses had the same competences as Austrian nurses due to the classification of their qualification. The interviewees consider information on the training content to be extremely important in order to be able to address the missing nursing skills in particular during induction. The interviewees described it as impossible to obtain this information directly from the migrant nurses during the induction phase due to the language barrier. In later conversations with the new immigrant colleagues about their training in their country of origin, the nurses interviewed were able to identify significant differences to nursing training.

One of the carers interviewed stated that he/she was of the opinion that immigrant carers lacked practical experience. This is particularly difficult in emergency situations and he/she emphasised the need for training measures in the area of emergency care because there are also differences in training here compared to the country of origin.

The interviewees described the use of carers with a migrant background who have completed their nursing training in Austria as an advantage due to their knowledge of the healthcare and nursing systems in both countries.

All of the carers surveyed identified major deficits with regard to care documentation. They stated that foreign carers do not understand the meaning of care documentation as it does not relate to medical parameters. Due to this lack of understanding, the interviewees have the impression that the immigrant colleagues have not focussed on the care documentation when familiarising themselves with it. However, they consider it particularly important to impart this knowledge and competence, as care documentation is not part of the training in the countries of origin. In everyday care work, the experts observe that the documentation of foreign carers is inadequate. They make fewer entries in the care report than their Austrian colleagues, which means that it is no longer possible to trace the residents' care progress. They also criticise the fact that some entries in the care report are not formulated clearly due to the lack of German language skills.

"Yes, it's very important. So that I can work well with the residents and, as I said, respond to their needs. And of course it would also be good if you could write care documentation in writing. (laughs) Because it's often a real guessing game. What does she mean now? What does it say now?" (IF, segment 18)

The interviewees criticised the lack of documentation of residents' health problems and the evaluation of interventions introduced. One of the carers interviewed stated that falls were not documented correctly by the migrant carers. To solve the problem of inadequate care documentation, she cited the joint support of the existing care team in order to increase the expertise of the foreign carers in this regard.

5.3 Assessing the professional quality of migrant carers

In the area of medical-therapeutic care, many of the interviewees did not recognise any deficits in the immigrant nursing staff. One of the interviewees stated that he/she could not recognise any competence with regard to qualifications. Another emphasised the need for control when applying ointments and administering medication. When it came to basic nursing care, all of them stated that the foreign carers had too few skills. This is also reflected in the statements made in the interviews about the lack of transfer of care-related information. Important information is not passed on, both in day-to-day care and during handovers. Regarding the handover of duties from the night shift by the new foreign colleagues, one of the interviewees stated that it is particularly often mentioned whether the residents have slept, but that there is no other information. In the area of care documentation, as already mentioned in Chapter 5.2, all caregivers interviewed emphasised the lack of competence of the immigrant caregivers. There were statements in all interviews about severe deficits in basic nursing care and hygiene.

*"...she does with the same wash-shoosh, what she did with Ol, because she cleaned down with Ol, she shaves dem by the mouth around each otherWhen you first
intimate area, then you'll have to take a second shot with you." (IB, Segment11)*

It was also criticised that foreign carers take too little time for basic care because they do not consider it important. One of the interviewees stated that he/she could not identify any differences in the quality of basic care between Austrian and migrant carers. Another interviewee expressed the view that the problem with conveying the lack of specialised knowledge in basic care is due to insufficient time resources for training.

Insufficient communication with the residents was a consistent tenor from the interviews on the question of professional quality. With regard to communication, however, one of the experts emphasised the advantage of multilingualism due to the increasing number of residents with a migration background.

"I think it's good that there are more and more foreign residents. Because I had a resident who only understood Bosnian. And as a carer, it's difficult for me to go there and interpret what she wants... And so it was really good to have a colleague on the team who could speak the language...." (IF, Segment20)

In the case of health complaints such as pain complained about by residents, one of the carers interviewed stated that their foreign colleagues do not react to this and rely on the existing carers to intervene.

In emergency care, it was uniformly expressed that the professional knowledge - especially in the treatment of falls - of the immigrant carers was good in this respect. One of the interviewees said that this could be expected of a qualified nurse, regardless of origin.

Two interviews revealed that running a care facility with migrant carers is conceivable and feasible. For a carer, the components of professional competence and humanity are a prerequisite. The second expert emphasised the possibility, but pointed out that care is reduced to essential activities.

5.4 Assuming responsibility in care

All interviewees particularly criticised the fact that foreign care staff do not react to residents' health complaints, such as pain complaints. They do not intervene in any way and do not pass the problem on to the qualified nurse. For example, one of the interviewees reported that, as a diplo- mised care worker in the main service, she sometimes receives no feedback from her foreign colleagues about falls suffered by residents. When she draws the attention of the responsible foreign employee to this, he/she receives the answer that the fall did not have any serious consequences. However, the qualified nurse interviewed emphasised that this behaviour varies depending on the origin of the foreign colleagues.

"Crashes or something like that, that they only reported in the evening, it flew once during the day and didn't happen and the next day there was a jolt, it was squeaky blue. So that's what I'm saying, there's no jerk message. You can't apply it to everyone, there are individual cases where this has happened. Many people say we do it ourselves, we know our way around anyway. It's not serious what happens anyway. But it's important as a graduate, the feedback." (IG, Segment14)

"...In this case of Bosnian/I believe Bosnian origin. That's happened a few times now. On the other hand, I've never experienced it with Tunisian origin." (IG, segment 16)

The interviewees stated that the foreign colleagues rely on the existing carers when residents have health or care problems. Especially when they are under time pressure, they simply pass on certain care measures. One of the carers interviewed said that basic care tasks were also neglected when the migrant carers had to work under time pressure.

As their understanding of care differs from that of existing carers, one of the interviewees said that he/she perceived a certain indifference on the part of foreign colleagues with regard to the performance of basic care tasks and that he/she lacked attentiveness to the needs of the residents. The core task of a carer, to support residents in the activities of daily living, is not fulfilled by migrant carers. All of the experts interviewed stated a lack of initiative on the part of their foreign colleagues. The flow of information fails because they agree in the affirmative when care-relevant points are passed on, but do not understand the actual content of the information. The interviewees consider it a failure on the part of their foreign colleagues not to enquire further. There were reports of emergency situations in which valuable time was lost due to this behaviour because existing carers relied on the fact that the foreign carer understood the information given and was expected to act correctly. One of the carers interviewed stated that emergency calls via the call bell system were not responded to at all. According to the carers interviewed, there were also no questions about resident care and general work processes. No questions were asked about care documentation either - which, as already mentioned in Chapter 5.2, is an unfamiliar type of documentation for the new immigrant carers. The interviewees stated that the foreign colleagues do not document the care measures and thus evade responsibility for their actions. One of the carers interviewed cited a lack of language skills on the part of immigrant carers as an excuse for inadequate documentation.

5.5 Familiarisation of the immigrant nursing staff

Some of the statements on the subject of induction vary greatly. The opinions of the interviewees differed particularly with regard to the induction period. All interviewees found the induction period for foreign carers to be challenging or even stressful.

Specialist content of the familiarisation

Here, too, there are different statements as to what content needs to be taught during the induction process. For example, one of the interviewees said that basic knowledge of nursing care should be a prerequisite for qualified carers. Others, on the other hand, emphasised that it is necessary to fully teach the basic content if the new immigrant nurses start work in Austria without practical experience due to the different training in their country of origin. This is important for understanding the holistic, person-centred care concept.

"It's like primary school. You have to explain everything, from A to Z, everything. ...There was training downstairs, but they didn't work in a nursing home or hospital." (IA, Segment6)

The carers interviewed cited knowledge of the resident's biography, preferences and habits, as well as medication and medical history, as particularly relevant content. One of the carers interviewed emphasised how important it was to know the residents by name. Dealing with medical emergencies was also mentioned as an important point for the familiarisation of foreign carers. In particular, information about the location of the emergency kit and the emergency numbers were emphasised by many. In terms of interdisciplinary cooperation, one of the interviewees stated that it was absolutely necessary to introduce GPs and therapists to the new foreign colleagues and to convey during induction that their information and instructions are important for nursing care.

The familiarisation period

As mentioned at the beginning, the opinions of the nurses surveyed on the familiarisation period for new immigrant colleagues are very ambivalent and range from a few days to three to four months. One of the experts, who has a migrant background herself/himself, believes that a period of a few days is sufficient for foreign carers and pointed out that getting to know the residents should be done on her/his own initiative. A longer familiarisation process only makes sense for residents with high and more medical-therapeutic care needs. According to him/her, rapid integration into the regular service and independent work is more successful in terms of learning than simply observing existing colleagues. Another of the nursing staff interviewed said that rapid integration into the regular service often arises out of the need to compensate for absences due to illness and said that this should be avoided. He/she also pointed out that there should be no criticism of the quality of nursing care if the new foreign colleagues have to work independently without sufficient familiarisation time.

All of the carers surveyed stated that the induction period depended on certain factors. For example, an adequate period for professional familiarisation was associated with professional experience, language skills, personality and the size of the care facility or the number of residents to be cared for. One of the interviewees stated that the familiarisation period depended on the origin of the foreign carer.

"Yes, I've noticed that the employees from the Balkans or Europe are totally different to those from the African continent or where they all come from. They are from the Balkans, they understand things faster, somehow...." (IA, Segment3)

When it came to familiarising themselves with the care documentation, all the care staff interviewed were of the opinion that they did not have enough time to do so.

The willingness of migrant carers to learn

In order to be able to work in the care sector in Austria, new immigrant carers must be prepared to expand their existing knowledge. All interviewees stated that this willingness is generally present among foreign nurses. In some cases, the new colleagues are very committed and endeavoured and require little guidance. One of the carers interviewed told us about a foreign colleague who is very intelligent and respectful when dealing with the residents and has the goal of working in Austria as a qualified carer. However, he/she raised concerns about their empathy skills.

For the carers interviewed, the efforts of the foreign carers are an important factor in the induction process. This requires learning from different existing carers and working methods. One of the interview participants said that the new immigrant colleagues do not all attach importance to learning from different carers and tend to carry out care at their own discretion once they have completed their induction.

"For example, I first started school in Bergwelt. I didn't like it at all. I said, [person] sorry, can we do it this way? Then she said, no, [person] taught me differently, I'll do it like [person]. Then I tell [person], you should learn from me and from [person]. Then at the end you can choose how you like...." (IA, Segment4)

The interviewees also see the willingness to learn in language acquisition, because the better the German language skills of the immigrant carers, the faster they are perceived to provide support.

All interviewees see personal initiative as an important indicator of familiarisation and a sign of interest in the nursing profession, but criticise - as already mentioned in Chapter 5.4 - that too few questions are asked. The tasks assigned are not clear if the information has not been understood. According to one carer interviewed, if there is initiative and interest in open questions, sufficient knowledge can be built up over 6 months. However, he/she sometimes perceives a certain indifference and says that no development is possible with a lack of interest. Personal initiative is also considered important when getting to know residents, doctors and therapists.

In order to work in the care profession in Austria, it is important for one of the interviewees that the immigrant carers adapt to the high standard of care, as the willingness to learn is related to the culture of the country of origin.

The operational readiness of foreign nursing staff

When it comes to covering services in the event of staff absences due to illness, all of the nurses interviewed reported that foreign nurses are very willing to step in at short notice and are perceived as providing great support in crises, especially during the COVID-19 pandemic or in the event of diarrhoea.

In everyday care work, many of the interviewees noted that migrant carers tend to neglect care when under high work pressure. In particular, personal care is not carried out sufficiently when time is tight. One of the carers interviewed reported complaints from foreign colleagues that there was not enough time and that care tasks were not completed. Work that is not completed has to be compensated for by the carers who are on duty the next day. He/she also complained about the neglect of communication.

"Yes, they always say there's no time, but we have enough, we certainly have time for laughter." (IA, Segment12)

Furthermore, two of the interview participants stated that the migrant carers do not take enough time for the life activity of eating and drinking. On the one hand, they complained that they did not pay enough attention to whether the residents had enough to eat and, on the other, that they acted quickly when it came to supporting the care recipients with their food intake. The interviewees reported residents complaining about the foreign carers because they did not comply with their wishes and certain care tasks, citing a lack of time as the reason.

One carer interviewed stated that there is no reaction from the immigrant colleagues to residents' health complaints, or that the solution to the problems is delegated to existing carers and they therefore have an "easier" job. The carer has the perception that foreign carers are only involved when it is a matter of achieving their personal goals. The fact that basic knowledge of general procedures and organisation is not yet mastered after months was also criticised.

The burden on existing carers during the induction process

The additional burden of the task of familiarising the foreign nurses was expressed by all the nurses interviewed. They emphasised the importance of teamwork for the induction process, but stated that it was nevertheless a challenge. They described increased mental strain due to the insufficient language skills of the migrant carers. The time it takes to gain an understanding of the German language is long and the high level of concentration required to carry out procedures and care for residents is described as very stressful.

"...As I said, it's often very difficult with foreign staff because they come and don't speak enough German. And then explaining everything simply takes much longer, is more time-consuming, more strenuous for us too. As we still have to continue with our programme or our work. And then it's a bit like that again (laughs) the heavy rucksack that you carry with you." (IF, Segment75)

Information has to be repeated several times and yet the transfer of care-relevant content is inadequate. When asked whether information has been understood, migrant carers often do not give an honest answer and there is no further opportunity for further explanations.

The concern for the residents is great when the foreign carers are not yet able to understand the specific needs due to the dialect. One of the interviewees stated that it was difficult to build trust and hand over responsibility. As an example, he/she mentioned the constant control and monitoring of medication selection and application. Another carer reported a lack of trust and stated that many care errors had occurred. It is also challenging to transfer trust in emergencies, especially as the foreign carers do not respond to emergency calls via the call bell system. According to all interviewees, there is also the time pressure of having to cope with everyday care work in addition to familiarising new colleagues.

Two of the interviewees stated that they perceived a lack of interest among their immigrant colleagues and that their explanations and information were not accepted by carers with academic training in their country of origin. They justify this statement by saying that their foreign colleagues do not listen to them, instructions are ignored and they react to instructions regarding correct hygienic working methods with rejection and resistance. A lack of critical faculties and a lack of understanding of the holistic care approach were also cited.

With regard to the motivation of migrant carers, one of the interviewees suggested that the reason for migrating to Austria was the better pay. One of the interviewees stated that he/she had not had any bad experiences when employing foreign carers. For him/her, there was no recognisable difference between Austrian and migrant carers during the induction process. He/she only described the fact of having to work in the regular care service alongside the induction as a challenging situation.

Suggestions from the interview participants for improving the familiarisation process

Despite all the critical comments, all the carers interviewed made suggestions for improving the induction process for migrant carers. Many emphasised that it is important to prepare foreign carers better. Particularly with regard to language skills, longer preparation and a check of their understanding of the content is necessary. Those responsible should not only rely on standard certificates, which are required as a legal prerequisite. One of the interviewees said that it would be necessary for foreign carers to complete a German course in Austria before starting work.

Two of the interviewees pointed out that foreign nurses need to be sufficiently informed about the field of nursing in Austria during the recruitment process.

Many said that the progress of skills acquisition requires continuous evaluation and that the induction period should be adjusted accordingly. Two of the interviewees mentioned familiarisation with the support of checklists and their adaptation to the professional integration process of foreign employees. All of the interviewees expressed that the initial familiarisation with basic care was necessary and that only experienced nursing staff from the existing team should be used for support.

5.6 Communication in the integration process of foreign carers

Communication in the integration process emerged as the most important category in the analysis of the interviews. There were by far the most statements on the topic of communication. The content discussed related to the nursing profession in general, communication within the team, business management, language acquisition and the burden of the language barrier between existing and new carers.

Communication in the nursing profession

The survey revealed that language is seen as the most important tool in the nursing profession and that learning German is essential in order to be able to work in nursing in Austria. Due to the language barrier, it is difficult for the nurses interviewed to convey the person-centred, holistic care concept. Foreign carers should be able to communicate specialist information.

"... Because a carer has to be able to tell me what's going on. If I don't understand him, if he says something biofc with / just understands the resident's name and coughs, you ask and he doesn't know what he's saying, that's just difficult..." (IG, Segment94)

One of the carers interviewed emphasised that understanding language is particularly important when caring for residents with dementia. In his/her opinion, it is not possible to compensate for language deficits with gestures and facial expressions in elderly people suffering from dementia.

Many of the carers interviewed described the lack of communication between their migrant colleagues and the residents, with key issues such as motivation and occupation falling by the wayside. One of the interviewees reported that he/she noticed more communication. According to one interviewee, the foreign carers argue that the lack of communication is due to a lack of time resources in day-to-day care. The interviewed carer refutes this view and states that communication is always possible during care activities in order to inform the residents and give them orientation. The carers interviewed stated that the new immigrant colleagues tend to simply affirm health complaints and needs expressed by the care recipients without further intervention due to the language deficit.

One of the participating carers expressed the idea that language is a special component for the acceptance of foreign carers by the residents. Understanding and recognising the elderly people being cared for increases this acceptance.

According to the interviewees, communication in an interdisciplinary context is avoided by foreign carers for fear of not being understood. All of the carers interviewed stated that the migrant colleagues communicate with each other in their native language in front of the residents as soon as none of the existing carers are present.

One of the experts interviewed cited the advantage of multilingualism for residents with a migration background.

Language acquisition

Many of the carers interviewed expressed that learning the local language is an essential part of the integration process, but that the German language is difficult to learn and that the time resources given to the immigrant carers are too limited. There was a consensus in the statements that the German language skills of the foreign colleagues should be sufficient to enable them to familiarise themselves with German and subsequently communicate with the residents and their relatives before starting work.

"Firstly, the language is very important. So you really need to have some knowledge of German right from the start. And that the induction is held in German as much as possible. Because then it's also with the residents and everything / at some point they have to be able to speak German, for our residents too and for the relatives..." (ID, Segment40)

In addition, good German language skills promote social integration into the team and the community of the care facility. In order to achieve this requirement, one of the interviewees expressed the idea of providing new immigrant nurses with language training in Austria before they start work and organising regular language courses in the care facility to further deepen and consolidate what they have learned. Some of the nurses interviewed pointed out that the learning progress of their foreign colleagues is individual and that communication is the best way to demand learning success. One of the interviewees also saw the responsibility for language acquisition with the management and said that deadlines should be set for learning success.

One of the interviewees also stated that when several immigrant carers from one country of origin are deployed, they communicate more in their native language, which delays the learning process.

The experts interviewed were willing to support the new immigrant carers in language acquisition, but stated that they failed due to a lack of knowledge about pedagogical approaches to teaching.

Communication within the team

All of the nursing staff interviewed emphasised difficulties in team communication with the new foreign colleagues due to the language and rated communication as inadequate. On the other hand, appropriate knowledge of German made it easier to work together. They stated that they had noticed that communication problems increase with a higher number of immigrant carers in the day care service. One of the interviewees expressed concerns that communication within the team would be lost altogether. The difficulty in trusting new foreign carers is therefore not due to their origin, but to a language deficit.

"Not trust, no. No, not at all, because a lot of things have happened. So it's not that when a new person comes, isn't it, that there's no trust because he's a foreigner, because I'm one myself, and so on, but it really has to do with the fact that they don't understand...." (IE, Segment61)

Many of the interviewees demanded that their immigrant colleagues be informed about their language skills, although one of the carers interviewed said that this would not prevent interpersonal problems. Multilingualism in the team is generally described as stressful and the wish was expressed that all carers on duty should speak German. One of the interviewed carers with a migrant background expressed her thoughts that foreign carers are very reluctant to communicate because they are inhibited by negative reactions from existing carers. It requires great concentration for the new colleagues to speak German and pass on information correctly. The problem of foreign carers' inhibitions to speak German was also described by another of the participating carers. He/she said that veteran colleagues in the care team should approach the migrant carers on their own initiative and offer support.

All of the experts interviewed described emergency situations as particularly challenging. According to one carer interviewed, life-threatening situations can arise due to the language deficits of the migrant carers. Here, too, there is the problem that the foreign colleagues answer in the affirmative despite not understanding the content of the information provided. In order to ensure a sustainable flow of information, it was expressed, as already mentioned, that the migrant carers must communicate if information was not understood.

The carers interviewed described the need to repeat information several times until the new carers understand the content as a particular burden. One of the interviewees raises concerns in this regard that the flow of speech of the existing carers when handing over the service further reduces their ability to grasp the content. In addition, the dialect in the country has an obstructive effect and instructions or information that are not understood are not carried out by the foreign carers as a result.

In the area of care documentation, the flow of information is interrupted by entries in the care report that are incomprehensible due to grammatical and spelling errors. One of the interviewees stated that they had observed that the foreign

carers sign off the planned measures in the care documentation without understanding the content.
One of the qualified nurses interviewed emphasised the importance of communication between the various professional groups in the team because they are dependent on feedback from the care assistants, who are in direct contact with the residents on a daily basis. The feedback is usually inadequate or incomprehensible due to the language deficit and the very limited vocabulary of the foreign colleagues. Some of the migrant carers do not pass on relevant nursing problems at all. The qualified nurse interviewed stated that the quality and frequency of feedback depends on the country of origin of the foreign carers.
One of the interviewees complained that there is no longer any dialogue within the team. He/she described discussions about stressful situations during breaks or after work as a kind of "supervision[11] for him/her. Due to the demarcation of foreign colleagues, these discussions no longer take place. Another interviewee pointed out that migrant carers also have no opportunity to talk about their personal problems due to the language barrier.
Some of the interviewees made suggestions for improving team communication. To promote communication, the team should be given the opportunity to familiarise their foreign colleagues with the dialect language through joint events outside of everyday nursing care. During the service transfers, there was a suggestion to schedule time for targeted preparation for the immigrant nursing staff in order to improve the outcome. The procedure in emergency situations and in the event of death should also be continuously communicated within the team outside of official meetings. The telephone emergency call should initially be made in English to take away the uncertainty of foreign colleagues and to avoid misunderstandings.
One of the care staff interviewed emphasised the advantage of multilingualism in relation to the care of residents with a migration background.
"Multilingualism is always good, I think. Arabic and French, for example. Well, now that we have more residents in geriatric care, we might get Muslims or something as old people in the future. That's why it's often not a bad thing if a certain number of them also work like that. So that they understand the language, because maybe they won't all be able to do that as they get older." (IB, segment18)

The communication of leadership in the communication process

All of the experts surveyed rated the communication of the management in the integration process of the new foreign nursing staff as inadequate. There were many critical statements, especially in the area of preliminary information. The interviewees emphasised the need to be informed about the language skills, the situation and the field of nursing in the country of origin, the training and qualifications, as well as the professional experience of the migrant nurses. One of the carers interviewed pointed out that it is not possible to assess skills without this information. This information is also seen as a prerequisite for providing migrant nurses with the skills that ensure a uniform level of knowledge across the entire care team. One of the interviewees stated that communication from management is extremely poor and that in some cases the team was not even informed of the day on which they would be starting work.

"Yes, in terms of information, we actually get relatively little, I have to say, yes? We often don't even know that a new employee is here. Where he's from. What qualifications does he have? So that's definitely not enough for us, and communication in general is where it starts again, isn't it? So that's definitely not enough for us, yes? We often have employees here, they're standing there and we often don't know, right, it has to be prepared in advance. " (IC, segment36)

The interviewees also expressed an interest in the background and social life of their new immigrant colleagues. For the entire integration process, all of the nurses interviewed expected more communication between the hierarchical levels and said that the management should also communicate directly with the foreign nurses. They expressed that the management is also responsible for providing linguistic support to the immigrant carers in the integration process in order to remove their inhibitions in communication. The need for existing nurses to communicate directly with management about the integration of new colleagues was also expressed by one of the experts interviewed. For the further recruitment of nursing staff from abroad, many of the participants called for the information provided by management regarding language skills to be based on understanding of the content rather than the certificates acquired. Furthermore, the suggestion of an information event for existing nurses and a translation of the induction concept into several languages was put forward.

According to the nursing staff interviewed, the introduction of the new immigrant colleagues should be accompanied by the nursing management of the respective nursing facility and the entire nursing team should be given the opportunity to exchange ideas outside of their professional environment.

5.7 Team development in the integration process of new foreign nursing staff

Although the integration of new immigrant nurses into the existing nursing team is a major challenge and leads to conflicts, the experts interviewed showed a great deal of empathy towards the new colleagues and offered ideas for solving the problems.

The empathy of the care team

The interviewees uniformly stated that it is difficult for new foreign carers at the beginning. The uncertainty of not knowing what to expect from their new colleagues in a foreign country, not knowing how to cope with everyday life, where to live in the future and how they will be received was described as stressful. Despite the challenge of having to adjust to a life that is very different from that in their country of origin, one of the carers interviewed, who has a migrant background herself/himself, said that it will not be difficult for the new foreign colleagues to feel at home in Austria.

The carers interviewed saw the language barrier in particular as a special challenge; they also rated German as a difficult language to learn. The interviewees showed a great deal of understanding in their statements because the foreign carers have to learn a new language, adapt to a new understanding of care and concentrate on the information provided by the existing carers. This is an enormous effort that is demanded of the new immigrant carers. One of the carers interviewed is of the opinion that no one takes into account the stresses and strains on foreign professionals, that they are separated from their families for months and are exploited for "our purposes". All of the interviewees therefore consider it important to create an environment in which the new foreign colleagues feel comfortable in order to be able to provide the required service. To this end, it is necessary to provide them with all the relevant information and to make all the resources available in preparation for the migrant nurses in order to make it easier for them to start work. The interviews revealed that existing carers try to put themselves in the shoes of their migrant colleagues and made a number of assumptions about their well-being. For example, one of the carers interviewed said that he/she suspected that the new colleagues were overwhelmed because they were under pressure to understand everything immediately and were perhaps afraid of losing their residence permit. Another of the carers interviewed told of a specific incident in which existing carers made fun of the pronunciation of a new foreign colleague during the handover of services. He/she made it clear that he/she found this behaviour unacceptable and that the foreign nursing staff needed to be supported by the existing nursing team. Another of the nurses interviewed emphasised the need for support and believes that long-serving colleagues in particular have a duty to support their new colleagues. Many of the interviewees stated that the existing carers are willing to support immigrant carers and expressed their sympathy.

The interviewees believe that the reason for the low level of communication with residents and colleagues of foreign carers is the language barrier and stated that this is why they do not talk about their own stresses and strains. In addition, the migrant carers were uncomfortable not being able to understand the basic principles after months on the job and may see themselves as a burden for the existing carers. The ex-persons interviewed expressed particular sympathy for the separation of foreign carers from their families. They try to show interest and are happy with their foreign colleagues when the families are able to travel to Austria.

"Like the one, she had two children downstairs, that's then / Yes. It makes you, how should I put it, sad yourself, but it's a long time until the children come up and that's terrible...." (IE, segment51)

One of the interviewees stated that he/she also embraces the new immigrant colleagues and offers them support. He/she went on to say that communication technology fortunately provides good opportunities for foreign employees to keep in touch with their families. In another care facility, one of the nursing staff interviewed reported with relief that the young immigrant colleagues had nevertheless settled in well and quickly.

Two of the interviewees pointed out that the foreign skilled workers had made a conscious decision to leave their home country and had to bear the consequences and knew that it would not be easy for them.

"I don't think it's easy for her, do you? I'll be honest. But by the way, you mustn't forget that you've decided to do this. You certainly don't make that decision overnight. I'm sure you're thinking about it, ge? I want to have something. And if I want something, then I also have to reckon with the consequences, that I have to take care of things myself, that I might not have it as easy as a Dasiger, ge?..." (IB, segment19)

One of these two carers interviewed expressed the idea that the colleagues who were approached were unable to empathise with residents or other carers in the team due to their own workload. One of the graduate nurses interviewed, who said that she had no negative experiences with any of her foreign colleagues, also reported very positively on the open welcoming culture of the management and emphasised the good support provided during the nostrification process, which the foreign colleagues would not be able to manage on their own.

Stresses and problems in the team

In this area too, the carers interviewed addressed the issue of language barriers and described multilingualism in the team as stressful. According to the interviewees, it is particularly difficult to pass on information and many expressed the need for all carers on duty to speak German. One of the participants expressed frustration that the foreign professionals leave certain tasks to the renowned carers. He/she cited care documentation as an example and explained the lack of assumption of responsibility by the immigrant colleagues. The different understanding of care was also expressed again in connection with the passing on of specific information on resident care. As already mentioned, the communication of migrant carers in their native language causes difficulties within the team.

"...Maybe anyway, because it's just a bit outrageous that they really speak in their mother tongue alongside the other employees." (IC, Segment27)

The interviewees stated that they felt aggrieved by this behaviour, but also expressed understanding that the foreign colleagues were better able to cope in this way. For several foreign carers in the day team, the interviewees expressed the feeling that they had to take responsibility for all professional matters. The graduate nurses interviewed reported the pressure of constant monitoring and the increased effort involved in handing over duties.

"Yes, it's a bit of a challenge for all my fellow graduates. Because you always check a bit more, see if it really fits. You also need more time in the handover." (ID, segment39)

Trust in the work of migrant carers was described by many as low. For example, the problem of dealing with a fall was again cited as inadequate. One of the interviewees even stated that she had to "catch up" with her foreign colleagues. According to the statements in the interviews, emergency care is also in the hands of the existing carers. In this context, one of the professionals interviewed emphasised that the emergency services must always be alerted by one of the existing carers. In a care facility with a residential area concept, the carer

interviewed described the concern for the residents if none of the existing colleagues are assigned to the residential areas. The interviewees attributed the lack of trust to the language barrier and pointed out that there was no connection with the origin of the migrant carers. An overwhelming majority of carers in the entire care team described the fear of losing their own values, understanding of care and humanity, as well as the feeling of being a stranger themselves. One of the carers interviewed, however, did not raise any concerns, with the exception of the worry that the German language would be neglected too much.
In order to maintain a good team environment, many of the participants emphasised that the existing nursing staff must also play their part. The need to treat foreign colleagues with courtesy and respect was mentioned. Giving them the impression that only the knowledge and behaviour of the existing nursing staff is valid should be avoided. Despite all efforts, it is not always possible to integrate all migrant nurses into the team, according to one of the nurses interviewed, who called for recognition for the additional work of existing colleagues in the familiarisation and integration processes.

Cohesion in the care team

The cohesion in the team with the integration of migrant carers was described differently by the interviewees. For example, one of the carers interviewed stated that the team spirit is good and that the new foreign colleagues can turn to the renowned employees at any time if they have problems. The high level of commitment shown by the foreign specialists when they were off duty was rated as particularly positive by one of the nurses interviewed and confirmed that this had strengthened the team spirit. However, the language barrier was again cited as a negative factor in this area, which, according to many of the interviewees, leads to group formations within the team. As a result, the feeling of being a community/team is lost. The different groups no longer approach each other.

"So it's also partly a case of us forming a kind of gretzel, yes. So really the Bosnians on the one hand, the Austrians on the other, that somehow a real team spirit never comes together, right? So I see that a bit under the main act, I say, right?" (IC, Segment25)

Many of the interviewees saw a deterioration in team cohesion and complained about the lack of support among each other. One of the experts interviewed reported negative reactions from existing carers when new foreign colleagues were to be trained. One of the participating diplomats rated the situation in the team as particularly bad and said that it was no longer a team. In her opinion, the reason for this lay in communication. Many of the carers interviewed gave examples of solutions to the complications in teamwork described. For example, all carers in the team at the facility should try to treat each other with courtesy. It was particularly important for one interviewee to convey to the foreign colleagues that they should offer support to the other carers on the day shift once they have completed their own tasks. Many of the caregivers interviewed emphasised the advantage of a mentoring programme for the new, immigrant caregivers in order to relieve the burden on the care facility's managers on the one hand and to avoid a feeling of disadvantage among the existing caregivers on the other. The management should communicate to the team that the foreign colleagues need more support due to the personal burden in the initial period. One of the nurses interviewed reported that this approach in her care facility required the understanding of the existing care team.

The conviction that it is always possible to be a team if all members deliver their performance was expressed by one of the graduates interviewed.

"...Because no matter where you come from, you can be a team. But, as I said, it still takes a little while to get there. From all sides, so not only from foreigners that they work, but also from our side, I have to say. Everyone has to contribute a bit to make it work." (IG, segment62)

5.8 The social integration of migrant carers

In addition to the professional integration of new immigrant carers, integration into the social community of the workplace and society is also important. The interviewees emphasised that the general conditions in Austria are much easier today than in the past, as the proportion of migrants is higher. It has become normal in society for people of different origins to live in Austria. According to an interviewed expert with a migrant background, it is easier to obtain a residence permit in Austria today than it was 30 years ago when he/she emigrated to Austria. He/she went on to say that the difficulties at the beginning were mainly language-related, but that social integration was easy. One of the interviewees praised the efforts of the management, which gave the new colleagues a lot of security by supporting them in their search for accommodation and dealing with the authorities.

Social integration in the professional environment

According to the interviewees, both sides are always responsible for successful social integration in the professional environment. Foreign carers not only provide their labour, they should also be able to participate in social life and be seen as part of the team by everyone in the care facility. One of the nurses interviewed emphasises the importance of the existing and foreign nurses in the team getting to know each other, but goes on to say that the immigrant colleagues should actively seek to integrate themselves. For example, the new foreign colleagues are expected to introduce themselves to everyone in their professional environment and inform them about their professional and language skills. Another of the carers interviewed said that they would be happy to provide support with social integration, but that the immigrant carers must be aware of their decision to migrate and the associated consequences. Many of the nurses interviewed believe that younger colleagues are more open and approach new immigrant carers without prejudice, but that they are very reserved at first. For their part, the renowned carers try to be unbiased and treat their new foreign colleagues with courtesy, but expect the same from them in return. Two of the interviewees stated that the majority of the existing carers were interested in the life, culture and past of the immigrant carers. Another interviewee stated that, conversely, their foreign colleagues had no interest in the history and culture of

Austria and that the motive for migration was purely monetary. There was agreement on the statement that the team spirit is lost when existing and newly immigrated carers withdraw into their respective social groups.

"...So really, as soon as there are two or three of them, then sometimes there is a kind of gretzel formation...Yes, so for me it's all a bit too little team spirit, I'd say. So one person doesn't approach the other and vice versa either." (IC, Segment42)

One of the carers interviewed emphasised that social connection is related to sympathy for a person and not to origin. This statement was confirmed by another of the interviewees, who said that the characteristics of individual personalities had more influence on social integration than origin. It was observed that foreign colleagues integrate at different speeds depending on their country of origin. Carers from the Balkans in particular were able to adapt quickly and make social connections. Despite the language barrier, some of the immigrant carers are able to integrate quickly into the social fabric of the care team, while others are very closed and the existing carers have problems accepting them. Many of the interviewees stated that gender roles in the countries of origin sometimes hinder social integration and that men find it easier to integrate than women. Another advantage is when foreign carers have already completed their training in Austria. All interviewees described the social integration of foreign carers as a labour-intensive process. Some of the experts reported a crisis in their own identity and a feeling of a loss of values due to the integration of several foreign colleagues into the team. One of the interviewees pointed out that with a majority of foreign carers in the team, there would be a kind of reversal effect and the existing Austrian colleagues would have to reintegrate. Once again, many of the experts interviewed cited the lack of language skills as a hurdle to social integration. When the migrant carers use the language skills they have learnt to communicate with their colleagues, this not only requires social integration, but also the deepening and consolidation of the German language. On the other hand, one of the carers interviewed stated that social integration in the professional environment fails when foreign professionals of their own origin communicate in their native language. The interviewees also believe that management is responsible for the success of the social integration process and can make a significant contribution to success by providing active support. It was stated here that immediate intervention by management is necessary if existing employees reject the foreign carers. The use of mentors as contact persons for the new immigrant colleagues to promote social integration was also mentioned by many. One of the nursing staff interviewed emphasised the advantage that a mentoring programme makes it possible to relieve the burden on management and that existing colleagues do not feel disadvantaged because the foreign nurses do not have to turn to the home or nursing service management with all their problems. He/she went on to say that the migrant carers should confide in the team and talk about their stresses and strains. With regard to the requirement of social integration, one of the carers interviewed suggested organising joint events in addition to official meetings in order to give the carers the opportunity to get to know each other better. Learning about the culture and needs of different nationalities is also an enriching experience for all carers. The experts interviewed stated that the same rules must apply to all carers in the team. One of the participants reported that the foreign colleagues were greeted with gifts. In his/her opinion, this approach had a negative impact on social integration and it would be better to invest this money in joint activities for the entire team.

"It would be great if they could just put a gift basket in the box for us and say: "Hey, for all of you. Because now we have a new employee. And so that you can get to know each other better, sit down and have a glass of champagne." For example...so that it's easier for everyone." (IF, Segment67)

According to the carers interviewed, the residents of the care facilities never reacted with rejection regarding the social integration of the foreign carers. Many of the interviewees stated that the carers were interested in the origin and personal history of their immigrant colleagues. In the area of interdisciplinary cooperation, more activity on the part of the foreign nursing staff would be desirable in order to establish contact with the therapists and doctors.

The immigrant carers' willingness to integrate

Only a few of the carers interviewed doubted their willingness to integrate. The motive for migrating to Austria was questioned in particular. One of the carers interviewed confirmed the assumption that many of the foreign professionals came to Austria because of the social system and that only a few appreciate the values of Western culture. The expectation that the infrastructure was provided by the state in accordance with the religious needs of the immigrant professionals was not correct. In the labour process, however, social integration is essential and a life based on religion in the country of origin is not possible. The interviewee questioned whether the foreign carers were willing to learn the German language. Some of the participants stated that some of their immigrant colleagues reject the person-centred, holistic approach to care in Austria because they cannot understand it. They emphasised that there is nevertheless a duty to adapt to the understanding of care, the good level of care, the structures and the time pressure.

"Every country has different cultures and they have to integrate into our culture. That was the most important thing. Because, whether Tunisians, Bosnians or whatever, everyone has a different approach to care. And they have to adapt to us, because it's a different system here. And when they've done that, that's integration for me." (IG, Segment68)

The interviewees expressed that the new, immigrant carers need to be aware of the importance of cultural and religious festivals in Austria.

Requirements for the successful social integration of foreign carers

According to the experts interviewed, the conditions for the successful social integration of new immigrant carers should already be taken into account during the preparation phase. When recruiting foreign carers, care should be taken to ensure that there is a willingness to socially adapt and an interest in life in Austria.

In order to better understand the needs of the residents, it is advantageous to familiarise oneself with the history and culture of Austria. One of the interviewees added that foreign care professionals who, in addition to their professional qualifications, also have respect and appreciation for the Austrian way of life are able to integrate socially more quickly. A suggestion for better preparation was made by another of the carers interviewed. The language acquisition for the recruited foreign carers should take place in Austria first and only then the professional integration. As justification, he/she cited the advantage that this approach could also impart knowledge about the culture in Austria.

5.9 The culture of migrant carers in the professional environment

During the interviews, the interviewees linked the behaviour of foreign carers to the culture of their country of origin. They revealed that the mentality is characterised by history and cultural differences. In particular, carers who immigrate from countries outside Europe have a different world view, according to the interviewees. Foreign colleagues' lack of knowledge about Austria's history affects the provision of care because they are not aware of what the generation that is now being cared for in long-term care has achieved. The immigrant carers lack a sense of belonging to the Austrian people and therefore a sense of responsibility for the residents. The carers interviewed stated that it was quite understandable that they did not feel as connected to the elderly people in the care facility. One of the interviewees raised the idea that there are certainly countries where old people are treated with a lot of respect. For another interviewee, it depends on the mentality as to whether the migrant carers perceive the residents as people and their needs. Many emphasised that if there is a willingness to integrate culturally, origin is irrelevant. However, the lack of adaptation to Austrian culture is seen as a fundamental problem.

Culture and behaviour of foreign nursing staff

According to the interviewed carers, foreign carers from Europe show a more open attitude than colleagues from other continents and are more likely to accept the professional expertise of existing carers. One of the interviewees reported an incident in which he/she pointed out to a foreign colleague the correct hygienic way of working when caring for a resident, which he/she then rejected in an angry manner. On the other hand, carers from the

Balkan region, who are very popular among the existing care team and immediately joined their colleagues. However, most of the foreign nurses are very reserved and many criticised the fact that the new colleagues did not introduce themselves. For example, one of the interviewees told us about a foreign carer who sat down in the duty room on the day he/she started work without introducing him/herself. It was therefore not possible for the care team to assign the new colleague. Many reported that the migrant nurses displayed behaviour that was unthinkable for Austrian nurses. Foreign carers have to be reminded several times to comply with rules that are a matter of course for existing carers. For example, one of the interviewees stated that it had happened in their care facility that migrant colleagues wore headphones on duty to listen to music or were

constantly approached on their private mobile phones.
"...yes, you have to tell them certain things more often. For example, that they shouldn't play on their mobile phones while on duty. Or to keep their AirPods in while they're working. That was something you had to say more often. " (ID, Segment52)
Another interviewee attributed the behaviour more to the personality of the individual foreign carers and said that good behaviour and friendliness cannot be learned, but must be brought along. With regard to induction, many of the interviewees raised the criticism that foreign professionals do not listen, seem convinced of their own knowledge and provide care at their own discretion without taking into account the person-centred care approach established in Austria. There were more and more statements that little interest was shown in care documentation in particular. The fact that foreign colleagues do not admit when they do not understand information is described as a fundamental problem. The existing carers rely on the assumption that the information passed on will be understood, so they rely on correct nursing follow-up actions and the frequency of errors increases as a result. This behaviour can lead to dangerous consequences for residents, especially in emergency situations. One of the interview participants raised the idea that this behaviour is related to the fear of annoying existing care staff by asking too many questions. One of the care assistants interviewed observed that migrant carers tend to leave care tasks to existing carers due to time pressure.

The behaviour of the foreign care staff in dealing with the residents

When interacting with the residents, all of the carers interviewed criticised the lack of communication on the part of the immigrant carers. The completely different understanding of care was also cited as a problem, as the foreign carers' lack of awareness of the residents' needs hindered relationship building. One carer interviewed said that the care recipients only accept the new, immigrant carers when they feel that they are perceived and understood. From a professional point of view, the understanding of care has an impact on care in the activities of daily life. One example given was that the migrant colleagues take too little time to feed the residents. The residents themselves show a fundamental interest in the new carers and are open to the culture and attitude they bring with them. The elderly are more open today and there is rarely rejection because of a carer's origin. They just sometimes seem surprised by the visual appearance if it differs from the Austrian carers. The interviewees stated that their foreign colleagues show little consideration for the residents and several reported that the immigrant carers listen to loud music while providing care. Sometimes in their own language. People suffering from dementia are particularly sensitive to this and suffer from this behaviour.

The subjective perception of existing carers with regard to the culture and behaviour of foreign carers

Many of the interviewees stated that they did not see a problem in the culture of the new, immigrant nurses and that cultural differences were not recognisable.

The areas in which the foreign colleagues show interest and which priorities they set depend on the cultural imprint. There were differences in the quality of the care provided by both Austrian and foreign carers.

"...It depends on the person. We've also had carers who say: "I don't do that." Or you've known that they don't wash properly. You can find that in every culture, whether it's ours or a foreign culture, it doesn't matter. So you find it everywhere. Either someone does it properly and knows their duties or they don't." (IG, Segment75)

One of the interviewees emphasised in their statements that their interest is more related to their understanding of care and that this makes it impossible for them to grasp the concept of holistic care. This is why the migrant carers place little value on the basic care of the residents. This lack of interest and lack of empathy lead to the existing carers turning away. One of the care assistants interviewed described the perception of indifference on the part of the immigrant carers and said that without empathy for the residents, it was inconceivable for him/her to work in the care profession. Many of the carers interviewed stated how important it is for their foreign colleagues to adapt to the care concept in Austria. Showing the residents respect and appreciation was essential in order to gain access to them. The interviewees stated that there is no bond between the immigrant carers and the residents. The affection that existing colleagues show to the carers is something that the interviewees feel is missing from the foreign professionals. Residents suffering from dementia in particular are sensitive and recognise whether friendliness is backed up by genuine appreciation for them as people. Some of the interviewees tried to explain their behaviour from the perspective of the attentive carers. They raised the assumption that behind the behaviour of their foreign colleagues is the pressure to do everything right in order not to lose their residence permit and that they are overwhelmed by the unfamiliar way of working. With regard to the aforementioned problem of not reporting back when information is not understood, one of the qualified nurses interviewed said that the immigrant nurses may have been inhibited and hoped that there would be no consequences. As the foreign carers in their care facility are very young, he/she also sees a connection with age and explained that similar behaviour can also be observed among young people from Eastern Europe. The only statements in the interviews that were directly linked to cultural imprinting related to gender differences. One of the interviewees questioned whether male carers, who are not allowed to care for female residents due to religious and cultural convictions, are suitable for practising the nursing profession in Austria. Secondly, concerns were raised that many of the residents are of faith and religion and that important values and traditions of our culture would be lost with a high proportion of foreign carers.

"Yes, since our generation is actually, yes, I almost dare to say, a bit religious, religion is very important and above all Catholic. I just imagine that if there are only more foreign carers, then there will be no Christmas. What are they supposed to do at Christmas then? They have no idea. Culture is a big problem in

my eyes, right? How that is actually, yes, part of life." (IB, segment29)
As a solution, the suggestion was made that the recruited nurses should be prepared for the culture in Austria in their country of origin and that cultural differences that have an impact on nursing care, such as dealing with dying and death, should be explained.

Culturally-orientated problems in the care team

The carers interviewed described problems in the care team due to the cultural imprint. When new foreign carers join the team, the existing colleagues are tense in advance. And although no major cultural differences to Austrian carers can be perceived, there is the problem that the new, immigrant carers sometimes do not show respect to their long-serving existing colleagues. Due to this behaviour, the interviewees say that they find it difficult to treat their foreign colleagues with empathy. One of the interviewees reported that some of the new carers do not adhere to the general rules of the team and the regulations of the care facility. They demand correct behaviour from the new foreign nurses and consequences from the management, but went on to say that the support of experienced nurses is also required in the event of cultural problems.

"...He does everything as he pleases, I think. He's always late for the handover or we always have to call him, we don't know if he's coming now, is he ill? We were there yesterday, too. I was there the day before yesterday. He comes on night duty at seven. That's not possible either. He has to say in advance whether he's coming or not, which I don't think is right for all of us. We're all making an effort, but he doesn't just turn up without an excuse, without anything sitting there. No reason, nothing! That's not possible either." (IA, Segment14)

Again, the problem was raised that migrant carers do not ask if they have difficulties understanding. In terms of everyday care, the interviewees expressed surprise that they do not obtain any information regarding food preparation in their foreign areas, such as the Austrian kitchen. This is incomprehensible to the interviewees, as they perceive the existing carers to be very patient with the uncertainties of their immigrant colleagues. As already mentioned in the previous chapters, the carers interviewed described the fact that foreign employees talk in their native language in their day-to-day work as a great burden and interpreted it as a lack of courtesy towards them. Concern was also expressed that foreign carers make arrangements with each other to provide care. Despite the sometimes very different cultural backgrounds, only a few of the challenges were described as a problem by the interviewees.

5.10 The role of leadership in the integration process

The statements of the nursing staff interviewed clearly expressed that the management and, subsequently, the home and care service managers in the individual care facilities bear significant responsibility for a successful integration process. Many of the interviewees said that they lacked targeted planning for the integration of new, immigrant carers.

According to the interviewees, the management's personnel policy has changed in recent years and it has decided to compensate for the staff shortage with foreign carers. One of the carers interviewed stated that the management was even relying on a predominant share of 90 percent foreign carers. For the interviewees, it would make more sense to recruit fewer but only well-qualified carers from abroad. In the recruitment process, special attention should be paid to the applicants' willingness to integrate and the likelihood of cultural adaptation in addition to their qualifications. According to the nursing staff interviewed, care service managers have little influence on the selection of applicants and personnel management in the care facility. They have to follow the guidelines of the management and integrate the foreign nursing staff assigned to them professionally and socially. If the professional qualification in practice and/or the integration fails due to the immigrant nurses' unwillingness, many of the interviewees believe that the management should keep the option open to terminate the employment contract and send the foreign nurses back to their home country.

For successful integration on a professional and social level, the implementation of an integration and familiarisation concept is essential for all of the nurses interviewed. One of the nurses interviewed suggested creating checklists in different languages for this purpose. The aim of the management must be to integrate the foreign specialists as quickly as possible. According to the interviewees, the company owner in particular fosters a very open culture of welcome. The management offers the immigrant carers support at any time if this is requested. They are initially provided with accommodation and are actively supported in their search for accommodation and the nostrification process. For the interviewees, this and the financial support are a basic prerequisite for the integration of their foreign colleagues, but in the interviews they criticised the lack of demands for language acquisition and the evaluation of progress in language skills. According to the interviewees, checking language skills is the responsibility of the respective nursing service managers. One of the care assistants interviewed cited the advantage of joint events to promote social integration and language acquisition. The language exchange also reduces the risk of foreign colleagues not being able to deepen their German language skills due to increased telephone calls with their relatives in their home country.

The carers interviewed stated that it was necessary for the integration process to invest in time resources in particular. In the interviews, they called for the foreign nurses to be accompanied by experienced nurses in the team, who only have to take care of the professional familiarisation and do not have to work in the regular service. Experienced colleagues should accompany the new carers over a longer period of time before they are given responsibility for a residential area. Many of the interviewees emphasised the need to deploy mentors from the existing care team in order to promote social integration into the community of the care facility. In addition, a mentoring programme offers the opportunity to relieve the burden on the house and care service managers, as the immigrant colleagues have an experienced carer as their first point of contact.

According to the interviewees, care home and nursing service managers play a significant role in the success of integration. It is therefore their responsibility to sensitise existing nursing staff who are reluctant to work with new immigrant colleagues by talking to them about the culture and way of life in their country of origin. Care home and nursing service managers should act as motivators when supporting foreign carers. It is the task of the nursing staff in service to support their immigrant colleagues in developing their understanding of nursing and to encourage them to expand their knowledge on their own initiative by asking questions when they have problems understanding.

"...They should listen to what I'm explaining now, or maybe take a bit with them and always ask. The most important thing is to ask. They shouldn't be ashamed or anything. They should just ask, maybe you should give them the confidence to do so." (IA, segment 11)

According to the interview partners, home and care service managers must familiarise foreign care staff with the infrastructure of the care facility, as well as the structural and procedural organisation, when they start work.

Passing on information by the management

The information passed on by the management was uniformly described by the interviewees as inadequate. The existing carers received very little information from the management about the newly arrived colleagues. They demanded that the management inform the care team about the training/qualifications, professional experience and German language skills of the foreign carers. The field of activity in the migrant carer's country of origin is also extremely important information so that the induction can be tailored accordingly. Existing carers in particular, who are entrusted with the induction, need more information.

"Nothing. It was only said that a lot of carers come from this place, otherwise none at all." (IE, Segment48)

According to the interviewees, the lack of information leads to a deficient view of the professional competences of foreign nursing staff. The interviewees also see the provision of information to new, immigrant carers as an important aspect of the integration process. Above all, the interviewees consider information about the field of nursing in Austria to be essential so that the new colleagues can realistically assess their professional activities. The responsibility for this task should be taken personally by the management so that the foreign carers also know who the company management is. Another important point mentioned by the carers interviewed was information and training with regard to cultural circumstances, such as the provision of food. Explaining the preparation and preparation of meals is a prerequisite for being able to guarantee resident care.

The care staff interviewed stated that the organisation of all work equipment must be guaranteed when they start work so that the new immigrant colleagues have a good start in their new professional environment. One of the graduate nurses interviewed reported that no work clothes had been prepared for the foreign carers on their first day at work, which meant that they could not be identified as carers by the residents and their relatives. All other work equipment such as the key or the access data for the care documentation software was also not

organised.
According to the interviewees, the management should continue to provide German courses and joint team events to consolidate and deepen the language skills of the foreign carers. Immigrant carers cannot be expected to introduce themselves to their colleagues on their own responsibility, as this is the task of the managers. This enables the entire team to form a solid basis for the integration of foreign carers.

The appreciation of existing carers

The interviewees criticised the appreciation of the existing nursing staff. The existing nursing staff feel burdened by the additional work of familiarising foreign nurses and stated that they do not receive any appreciation for this from the management. All colleagues are treated equally, regardless of their company affiliation. As a result, the employees of the existing care team feel that their experience is not valued, which explains the lack of respect shown to them by their foreign colleagues. The increasing number of immigrant nurses reinforced the feeling that the work, expertise and experience of the veteran nurses was losing value. According to the interviewees, praise and recognition for the existing care team are important in order to minimise the feeling that the focus is on the performance of foreign carers.

"...But what I would like to see (...) is that the existing employees are not forgotten. Because it's also a task for us and it's exhausting to explain everything to someone, to train them and so on. And it would also be nice to see a little more recognition of the existing life or the integrated colleagues. That you simply say: "Thank you for taking the time now." Or, yes, even if it's a small gift. It doesn't have to be anything big. But once / far from it, a thank you and something like that: "Thank you, you've done so much for them and you've been there for them and that has encouraged them so much. " That would have been nice once. So it's not just the foreign staff who are always being raised to the heights, but also the existing staff. (IF, Segment54)

One of the graduate nurses interviewed complained about the inadequate offboarding process in order to find out the reasons for existing nurses leaving the company and subsequently to be able to derive measures to increase employee satisfaction.

Management errors in the integration process

Many of the interviewees reported management errors in the ongoing integration process. In particular, the limited time resources for induction and the lack of information were emphasised by the carers interviewed. One of the interviewees was upset that the managers did not have the right to criticise the quality of care if neither the time resources nor the information were provided sufficiently. Due to the lack of information, the existing nursing staff associated certain competences with the qualifications of the foreign nursing staff. As the area of activity of the immigrant colleagues in their country of origin differs greatly from that in Austria, they were unable to fulfil the expectations of the care team. This led to unrest and dissatisfaction among the existing carers.

One of the interviewees complained about the failure of the management to define clear contact partners (mentors), so that the foreign colleagues turn to the home or care service management with all their concerns. The existing carers felt disadvantaged by the increased commitment of the home management, even though the team had warmly welcomed the immigrant carers.

"Yes, they gave them a very warm welcome, I have to say. Yes, some of them were perhaps a little too involved, especially the head of the home, who / I mean, of course they have the whole family in another country. And he really struggled to get them into a flat, to get them a bit closer to the team, which was a great fit anyway. But yes, he's still being approached by a Tunisian woman and he keeps going back to the office. And yes, so maybe you draw the line a bit more..." (ID, segment37)

"...Now it's better again, but a few months ago it was a thing that they all felt disadvantaged..." (ID, Segment38)

The fact that the management had not obtained any feedback from the existing nursing staff regarding progress in language skills was also criticised. In addition, it was not possible to make suggestions for improving the integration process.

Welcome gifts organised by the home and care service managers for the new foreign carers caused particular unrest. The existing carers felt that they were being disadvantaged by this and wanted to invest in joint team events.

One of the care assistants interviewed stated that the management did not provide any support to the existing employees in the integration process.

5.11 The integration of foreign carers as a relief for the existing care team

The aim of recruiting nursing staff from abroad to reduce the workload for the company's nursing staff, reduce the workload and increase the quality of care can certainly be recognised in the interview statements. For example, the interviewees stated that the deployment of migrant nursing staff was perceived as positive. The quantitative increase in personnel is described as an advantage, as the foreign colleagues work full-time and this reduces the workload. In addition, the professional expertise that the immigrant colleagues bring with them is described as valuable. One of the interviewees said that you have to be grateful for the support. Without the labour of immigrant carers, care in Austria could no longer be maintained, said another interviewee. The interviewees stated that the willingness of the new foreign carers to work is high and that they are prepared to take over missing services in the event of staff absences due to illness. In addition, the immigrant carers can help to compensate for the additional workload during the induction phase when staff are absent.

The interviewees said that the willingness of foreign carers to take on duties during the Christmas period because the Christian holidays have no significance for them is greatly appreciated by the existing carers. This results in significant advantages in the organisation of the duty rota.

"So one advantage I've noticed is that it's Christmas time and all that, yes? Because they just don't celebrate Christmas now, right? They simply organise

their employees during the Christmas period. It always depends, that always goes down well. Some people volunteer to say: "Yes, hello, we're celebrating, I don't know, no Christmas on the 24th, you could organise a shift for me. " So that's a positive thing." (IC, Segment6)

As already mentioned, many emphasised the advantages of multilingualism in the team. Especially against the background of an increasing number of migrants in Austria who have to be cared for in care facilities in old age. This facilitates communication with the residents, who can express their needs more easily in their native language. The interviewees see multilingualism as a valuable resource, especially with regard to biographical work and dementia among residents of foreign origin. In this way, understanding can be gained for the behaviour of residents with a migration background and a relationship can be established.

5.12 Summary of the results

The use of foreign carers to compensate for the shortage of skilled workers was generally viewed positively by the interviewees. However, two of the interviewees expressed strong reservations as to whether the solution approach was suitable for recruiting foreign carers. They justified this with the assumption that the motive for immigrant carers to come to Austria was to gain access to the good social system. From a professional point of view, the nurses interviewed emphasised that although their foreign colleagues brought with them a great deal of knowledge in the field of medical and surgical care, they had major skills deficits in basic care. This was repeatedly evident in the analysis of the interviews in many categories and leads to major problems in everyday nursing care. The prevailing concept of person-centred, holistic care in Austria is alien to the immigrant carers and teaching them to understand this is a particular challenge for the existing carers. The familiarisation of the foreign colleagues was described as correspondingly challenging. Communication is also particularly difficult for the interviewees. This relates both to communication within the care team and with the residents and has an impact on cooperation, team development and the quality of care. It is not only the language barrier that poses a challenge here, but also the transfer of information. The flow of professional information within the team comes to a standstill as the foreign carers do not pass on care-relevant information or only do so inadequately. The fact that multilingualism in the team leads to the formation of groups was described as a burden. Immigrant colleagues with the same mother tongue and Austrian carers withdraw into their respective social groups. This leads to a split in the team and makes collaboration more difficult. In particular, the fact that foreign carers talk in their native language in the presence of existing carers is perceived as stressful. Nevertheless, many experts expressed that multilingualism in the team is also a valuable resource because it can improve the quality of care for residents with a migration background. Cultural

Differences are mainly associated with the behaviour of foreign caregivers. According to the interviewees, some of the migrant carers do not adhere to formal

or informal rules and this causes unrest in the care team. However, many of the interviewees expressed their understanding and suspected inhibitions due to language deficits and insecurity behind the behaviour.
The nurses interviewed see the responsibility for the success of the integration process of the new immigrant colleagues primarily with the management. Many of the challenges and problems encountered are due to the lack of preparation for the integration process, as well as the support and information provided to the existing nursing team and the foreign nurses. Information about the training, professional experience, previous field of activity in the country of origin and actual language skills are essential in order to be able to adequately familiarise the foreign carers. During the induction phase, all interviewees criticised the shortage of time resources. More space should also be given to social integration into the care team. The entire process must be adapted accordingly by the management, whereby the interviewees made many suggestions for improvement.
Despite the many challenges, the feeling of relief through the deployment of migrant carers was described in the interviews.

6 Discussion

The results from the interview analysis are consistent with previous findings described in other research or literature on the topic. It is striking that in many areas the perspective of existing carers, who play an essential role in the integration process of migrant carers, is not taken into account in the literature. These findings are at the forefront of this study and thus complement the body of knowledge on the topic.

In the literature, the **integration of foreign nursing staff is** justified with facts and figures **as a solution to** compensate for the staff shortage. For example, the update of the personnel requirements forecast by Gesundheit Osterreich GmbH predicts a need for around 200,000 nurses by 2050. (Juraszovich et al., 2023)

Another reason, according to Goldgruber (2023), is the general development of worldwide migration due to social and political crises and globalisation. (Goldgruber et al., 2023)

Faupel and Weiner (2023) even describe the recruitment of foreign nursing professionals as having no alternative because the labour market in German-speaking countries has almost run out of nurses. (Faupel & Weiner, 2023)

The results of this study show a more complex picture, because although the interviewees view the approach of integrating foreign carers positively, it is not seen as a solution to the shortage of skilled workers. The interviewees consider investment in making the care profession more attractive with better pay and the expansion of home care to be the solution. They also associate the integration of migrant carers with the additional effort of familiarisation, language problems and a different self-image for care.

The problem of the different **understanding of nursing care between** native and foreign nursing professionals is described in detail in the literature reviewed. With holistic nursing care, immigrant nurses are confronted with a completely different view of the nursing profession. (Faupel & Weiner, 2023)

The cooperation between care professionals, for whom the person-centred, holistic care approach is part of their professional identity, and colleagues who see care as a medical-technical profession is described as difficult. This is mainly because the operators of the care facilities assume that the migrant nurses assume the professional identity of the local nurses and ignore the differently defined professionalism of the foreign employees. (Bossle & Kunhardt, 2022)

The explanation lies in the training of migrant carers, many of whom have an academic degree and are highly qualified. (Faupel & Weiner, 2023) It was repeatedly mentioned in the interviews that basic care, communication and the needs of the residents are not important to the migrant carers and that this puts a strain on them. This can be attributed to the differentiated understanding of the nursing profession and has not yet been described in this clarity in other studies.

If we look at the deployment of foreign nursing staff in other countries, we see a significant difference to the present study and the area of deployment in long-term care. For example, the area of deployment after recruitment in the USA, which employs a high proportion of migrants in the care sector, differs significantly from that in Austria. The majority of foreign nurses in the United States work in intensive care, surgery or in the operating theatre. (Shaffer et al., 2022)

The deployment of foreign carers in long-term care is more difficult, as a high proportion of basic care has to be provided here. The wish to initially deploy the immigrant carers in basic care and thus minimise difficulties in assuming responsibility cannot therefore be confirmed. This is also reflected in the interviews. The interviewees expressed their astonishment that the immigrant colleagues have a lot of knowledge and skills in the medical-technical areas, but are not able to perform simple basic care tasks, such as personal hygiene, correctly.

This clearly shows the deficient view of the existing carers due to the deployment of foreign professionals in long-term care. Their strengths and knowledge cannot be utilised by the immigrant carers. (Faupel & Weiner, 2023)

In this respect, the deployment of foreign specialists in long-term care should be reconsidered and the training content and field of activity in the country of origin should be taken into account during recruitment.

The lack of willingness on the part of immigrant carers **to take responsibility**, which was often criticised in the interviews, is not described in the literature reviewed. This leads to the assumption that the behaviour of the foreign carers described by the interviewees of leaving the responsibility for certain care activities to their Austrian or veteran colleagues is a misinterpretation of the existing carers or that the perspective of the existing carers has not yet been taken into account in the literature. The reason for shifting responsibility may therefore also lie in a lack of ability to express oneself linguistically.

Communication is cited in all literature sources as an important indicator for the success of the integration process. The results of the interviews confirm the extensive discussion of communication in the integration process in the literature, as the communication category received the most statements. However, the nurses interviewed not only commented on the language skills of their foreign colleagues, but also referred to communication within the team, with the management and the burden on the existing nurses with multilingualism in the team.

The profession of healthcare and nursing requires a high level of communicative competence, not only in the professional exchange with colleagues and in the interdisciplinary team. Communication with residents in particular is an essential part of nursing care. (Moser, 2010)

All of the carers interviewed stated that the immigrant carers lacked language skills. The lack of communication with residents in particular was often cited, as this represents an indicator of good care quality for the existing carers - in connection with holistic care. Communication within the team and the passing on of care-relevant information was also rated as deficient by the interviewees. Many of them described the fact that the foreign nursing staff nevertheless answered in the affirmative when there were difficulties in understanding as very problematic.

In addition to the language deficit, some of the interviewees suspected other obstacles such as inhibitions about expressing themselves incorrectly or fear of being exposed because they still do not understand information or its content after months.

Bossle and Kunart (2022) state that it is not only language skills that play a role, but also the type of communication, which is influenced by both the culture and the values of the immigrant carers. (Bossle & Kunhardt, 2022)

It therefore does not seem right to base communication purely on language acquisition. However, the interviewees stated that assessing language skills solely on the basis of legally required language certificates does not seem right.

Faupel and Weiner (2023) also describe this, stating that the language skills of foreign carers are very heterogeneous despite a uniform language level. (Faupel & Weiner, 2023)

Accordingly, the interviewees described the **familiarisation** of the new immigrant carers as difficult. The fact that information has to be repeated several times and that there is still no certainty of understanding was described as a burden. Although the information about an adequate familiarisation period varied, many found that the time resources were too short.

This is also confirmed by the results of the TransCareKult project in the IG Landesnetzwerk Hessen. It is noted here that the familiarisation process takes place "on the job" and that the day-to-day work of the caregivers providing the training also has to be managed on the side. (Gold et al., 2019)

The additional task of familiarisation was described by the interviewees as demanding and challenging, and is an achievement of the existing carers that should not be underestimated.

According to Gold et al. (2019), the induction of new immigrant carers is even perceived as a "punishment", as it requires a lot of time resources. (Gold et al., 2019)

This problem was also expressed by the nursing staff interviewed. Accordingly, time off from the regular service to familiarise the new foreign colleagues was considered useful. A lack of initiative on the part of the immigrant carers was also mentioned in the surveys. The existing carers expect the new colleagues to ask specific questions. If these expectations are not met, the existing carers interpret this as a lack of interest in the nursing profession.

Personal initiative is also described in the literature as an indicator for recognising foreign carers. There is a strong correlation between the initiative of foreign carers and their recognition as a person and professional by the existing care team. (Gold et al., 2019)

In the interviews, many statements were made about the willingness to learn and commitment during training. Nothing could be found on this topic in the literature reviewed.

There are many chapters in the literature on the topic of **social integration**, **team development** and the challenges of cooperation between different **cultures**, which in turn are described in connection with communication and the understanding of nursing. Nothing of this kind is explicitly mentioned in the literature with regard to the statements made by the nurses surveyed about the difficulties they experience in the team and the expression of empathy that the existing nurses show towards their new immigrant colleagues.

Nevertheless, the area of culture and cultural sensitivity is described in detail. In their book, Bossle and Kunart (2022) cited the variant of multiculturalism, which presupposes subordination to the dominant culture in order to avoid conflicts within the care team. This is characterised by the fear of losing one's own values and cultural characteristics. (Bossle & Kunhardt, 2022)

This fear can be seen in the statements of the interviewees as well as in the described behaviour of the migrant care workers.

Faupel and Weiner (2023) emphasise the importance of strengthening the team culture by requiring intercultural skills and go on to say that integration fails due to the frustration of the care team. Training measures on cultural sensitivity should prevent this and they see the management level as being responsible (Faupel & Weiner, 2023)

The study on the TransCareKult project, on the other hand, describes the limits of **management's** ability to influence the integration process and states that middle management in the form of ward managers can still have the greatest impact here. Nevertheless, the success of the social integration of foreign nursing staff always depends on the individual persons and their attitude. (Gold et al., 2019)

This thesis is best reflected in the interviewees' statements, as they describe individual behaviours of the immigrant nurses that appear to hinder social integration. With regard to the behaviour of the existing carers, situations were also described such as mocking or laughing at their foreign colleagues due to the incorrect pronunciation or expression of the German language. One of the nurses interviewed took sides with the immigrant nurses and criticised their colleagues' behaviour.

The TransCareKult study also describes a range of behaviour on the part of existing carers, from disrespectful to respectful. Nurses who treat their new, immigrant colleagues with respect rarely give any indication of the behaviour of those who act disrespectfully. (Gold et al., 2019)

Examples of the role of **management** in the integration process were found in some of the academic articles in the literature reviewed. Many statements were made in the interviews and a great deal of responsibility for the integration process was attributed to both the management and the managers in the care facilities.

One of the articles describes the integration of foreign nursing staff as a change management process that requires more than just adapting the nursing profession. The corporate culture and structures must also be adapted. All affected employees must be involved in the process in order to achieve a positive attitude towards the integration process. This includes good preparation to strengthen intercultural competences and a well-thought-out integration concept. (Faupel & Weiner, 2023)

Angelovski (2014) cites the need to not limit integration training to care alone, but to include communication, encounters and cooperation between people of different origins. (Angelovski, 2014)

According to the interviewees, there was no preparation for the integration process on the part of the management. One particular criticism was that they did not receive any information about their new, immigrant colleagues. The interviewees also felt there was a lack of accompanying support for the foreign nursing staff in terms of language development. The interviews clearly showed that the foreign nurses also need to be prepared for the culture in Austria, the understanding of nursing and the new field of activity.

This statement is echoed in the literature, which emphasises the importance of incorporating cultural aspects into the preparation of foreign carers. (Goldgruber et al., 2023)

The interviewees' request to appoint mentors for the new immigrant colleagues and the desire to organise joint activities with the entire team is also described in the literature as beneficial. (Faupel & Weiner, 2023)

In their statements, all of the carers interviewed emphasised the importance of valuing the existing care team and stated that they felt that the foundation was focusing on the immigrant carers. No concrete information on this could be found in the literature. The critical comments of the interviewees are closely related to the integration concept and the extent to which all components of the integration process were considered. If the integration process is planned and well prepared, as described in the literature, it is highly likely that many problems could be avoided.

Faupel and Weiner (2023) aptly describe the integration process as a joint task for all individuals involved and go on to explain that the adaptation of structures and processes, as well as the utilisation of expertise, is necessary in order to be successful. The human factor should always be taken into account. (Faupel & Weiner, 2023)

This statement can be derived from the results of the interviews, as the interviewees made many suggestions for improving the integration process. However, they complained that they did not have the opportunity to actively participate.

7 Limitations

As resources are limited within the scope of a master's thesis and only 7 interviews were conducted, this must be considered a limitation. In addition, the field of research is limited to the care facilities of one operator, which restricts the perspective of the interviewees. The circumstances related to the organisation of the integration process only refer to facilities of one company, although this is a case design and the results can be generalised to similar cases. As the author works as a manager in the company, this presumably had an impact on the conduct of the interviews and the analyses. The recruitment process was not able to reach existing nursing staff with experience in integrating foreign colleagues from all of the organisation's care facilities. Nevertheless, the recruitment strategy was suitable for recruiting sufficient participants, the influx of interested parties was good and the interviews were informative. A saturation of the data was achieved in the analysis. Triangulation must be considered to a limited extent for the good criteria, as the analysis of the data from the interviews was kept simple and only subjected to categorisation. The results were made available to the interviewees for communicative validation. In their feedback, the interviewees stated that the problems of the integration process were well understood. No further steps in the validation process were planned. Including foreign carers from the group of companies in the survey was not the aim of the present study; reference can be made to further research in the outlook.

8 Conclusions

The results of the surveys lead to the conclusion that existing carers are basically positive about the integration of foreign carers. The burdens and challenges they describe being confronted with on a daily basis are closely linked to the information and preparation of existing and migrant carers for the integration process. The assumption that it is enough to recruit skilled workers from abroad and support them in their search for accommodation and the nostrification process is fundamentally wrong. In order to successfully organise integration on both a professional and social level, it is necessary to deal with all components of integration in advance and to involve all individuals involved. The suggestions for improvement made in the interviews are a valuable resource that can be utilised. A well thought-out integration concept can be developed on the basis of this discussion. Its implementation requires ongoing evaluation and adaptation to the individual situation in the care facilities. The existing carers are one of the most important groups in the integration process, as it is up to them to implement the integration measures in practice. The burdens and challenges described in the interviews can be avoided or minimised through good preparation, information and measures to raise awareness. Sufficient information about the origin, culture and motives of foreign carers migrating to Austria can help to reduce prejudices. Information about the training content, the field of activity, the professional experience and the nursing understanding of the future colleagues are essential points so that the existing carers can adapt to the integration. However, it is not their task to define the content of the induction programme. The responsibility for the content of the induction concept clearly lies with the management and should form part of the integration concept. A good induction concept, adapted to the needs of the foreign carers, is a guideline to which the carers who are entrusted with the induction can orientate themselves. This relieves the burden on existing carers and reduces pressure. During the preparation phase, it is necessary to take a close look at the foreign carers' understanding of care, as well as the person-centred approach to care in Austria. It is a particularly challenging task to convey an understanding of the different perceptions of the nursing profession. The attitude of immigrant carers towards the nursing profession as a profession that requires an objective approach to the challenges of everyday care is often misinterpreted by existing carers as a lack of interest. In long-term care in particular, relationships also develop on an emotional level between residents and carers, which makes it difficult to draw personal boundaries. In addition, basic nursing care in the countries of origin of foreign professionals is usually provided by relatives. When migrant carers are confronted with basic care tasks, they feel that their skills are being denied. Accordingly, it is also essential to prepare foreign carers for the new field of activity and the nursing profession in Austria. In addition to language skills, they must be trained on a professional and social level before they are integrated into the nursing service. Middle managers have a particularly important role to play in the integration process. They are the point of contact for existing and immigrant carers and must accompany the integration process with a great deal of knowledge, empathy and solution-orientation. In addition to professional, social and culturally sensitive training, care home and nursing service managers must receive special training in team development in order to recognise problems in the team and, if necessary, take swift action to counteract escalation. The management is responsible for developing a tangible integration concept that covers all the areas mentioned. For the successful, long-term and sustainable integration of foreign nursing staff, it is necessary to invest in time and financial resources. In addition, the existing nursing staff must be recognised for the additional work of training and integration, otherwise there is a risk of losing these valuable employees. With these measures, many challenging situations can be avoided and integration can be made easier for both existing and migrant carers. Further research was also carried out into other care facilities run by other operators and whether the results can also be transferred to the acute setting of a hospital. Research into the use of participatory, culturally sensitive methods with new foreign and existing nursing staff also provided valuable results for improving the quality of integration processes.

9 Bibliography and list of sources

Angelovski, I. (2014). Driving colourful teams. *Pflegezeitschrift, Vol. 67, Issue 2,* 108-111.

Bachinger, N. (2009). *From the multicultural to the transcultural care team.* Dr Muller.

Bachmann, A., & Wolf, J. (2007). Leading multicultural teams: A conceptualisation and empirical analysis of the need for different leadership styles. *The Journal of Business Economics*, *77*(10), 1035-1064.

Bettig, U., Frommelt, M., & Schmidt, R. (2012). *Fachkraftemangel in der Pflege: Konzepte, Strategien, Losungen*. medhochzwei Verlag.

Bonacker, M., & Geiger, G. (2021). *Migration in care: how diversity and individualisation are changing care*. Springer.

Bossle, M., & Kunhardt, H. (2022). *Integration of foreign employees in nursing care: Theories, concepts and pedagogical experiences and framework recommendations for practice*. Hogrefe AG.

Dewes, A. (2022). Procedures for anonymisation and pseudonymisation of data. In *Data economy and data technology: How value is created from data* (pp. 183201). Springer.

Dresing, T., & Pehl, T. (2015). *Praxisbuch Interview, Transkription & Analyse: Anleitungen und Regelsysteme fur qualitativ Forschende*. dr dresing & pehl GmbH.

Ertl, A., Benfer, A., Bychowski, U., Gehlen, L., Geiger, I., Pickel, I., Spahn, C., Gulec, A., Angel-Cubillo, F., Becker-Reuter, M., Grieger, D., Demirci, S., Kraus, B., Zanier, G., Baric-Budel, D., Al Baghouti, G., Taspunar, F., Artmeyer, A., Kloos, E., . . . Foitzik, A. (2022). For culturally sensitive elderly care. A handout. In.

Faupel, A., & Weiner, T. (2023). Integration of international nursing staff. How intercultural teamwork succeeds. *Thieme CNE Nursing Management*, *16*, 2-16.

Fent, T., Furnkranz-Prskawetz, A., Hammer, B., & Danhel, G. (2019). Demographic change-changed framework conditions for the welfare state?

Feustel, R. (2021). *Deduction and induction*. University of Leipzig. Retrieved 20.04.2024 from https://home.uni-leipzig.de/methodenportal/deduktion_induktion/

Flick, U., von Karkoff, E., & Steinke, I. (2009). *Qualitative research: A handbook.* Rowohlt.

Gleitsmann, M., Graser, G., Linder, A., Meissner, P., Mittelbock, H., Sengschmid, E., Zalesak, M., & Zanol, A. (2022). *Analysis of the skilled labour potential of migrants in Austria*.

Gold, C., Smeaton, S., Maliki, S., Tersch, M., & Schulze, U. (2019). An undercooled welcome culture. Results of a qualitative study on the situation of newly immigrated carers in inpatient facilities. *Pflegewissenschaft- Zeitschrift fur Pflege, Pflegeforschung, Pflegepraxis und Pflegemanagement*, *22*(3/4), 130-141.

Goldgruber, J., Dohr, S., & Hartinger, G. (2023). Migration-Challenge and opportunity for the future of nursing care. *ProCare*, *28*(3), 52-55.

Hahn, S. (2023). *Historical migration research*. Campus Verlag.

Herlach, S. (2021). Welcome to Germany. *CNE Nursing Management*, *8*(04), 4-11.
Fulda University of Applied Sciences. (2020a). *Country dossier Bosnia and Herzegovina*. Retrieved 07.01.2024 from https://www.hs-fulda.de/fileadmin/user_upload/RIGL/IntIP/Country_dossier_Bosnia_and_Herzegovina.pdf
Fulda University of Applied Sciences. (2020b). *Country dossier Republic of the Philippines*. Retrieved 07.01.2024 from https://www.hs-fulda.de/fileadmin/user_upload/RIGL/IntIP/Laenderdossier_Philippines.pdf
Holzweber, L., Pilwarsch, J., Zach, M., Grubock, A., Mathis-Edenhofer, S., & Wallner, A. (2022). Annual report health professions register 2021.
Hormel, U., & Scherr, A. (2010). *Discrimination*. Springer.
Janssens, U., Addo, M. M., & von Bergwelt-Baildon, M. (2022). The COVID-19 pandemic-an epochal event. *DMW-Deutsche Medizinische Wochenschrift, 147*(20), 1297-1298.
Juraszovich, B., Rappold, E., & Gyimesi, M. (2023). Nursing staff forecast. Update to 2050. update of the nursing staff requirement forecast 2030. results report.
Kline, D. S. (2003). Push and pull factors in international nurse migration. *Journal of nursing scholarship*, *35*(2), 107-111.
Krings, T. (2013). From "Foreign Employment" to the Red-White-Red Card: Social Partnership and Migration Policy in Austria. *Austrian Journal of Political Science*, *42*(3), 263-278.
Kuckartz, U. (2018). *Qualitative content analysis. Methods, practice, computer support, 4th ed*. Beltz Juventa.
Lenhart, M. B. (2018). *Care worker migration to Austria: an empirical analysis*. Peter Lang International Academic Publishers.
Mayer, H. (2022). *Applying nursing research: Elemente und Basiswissen fur Studium und Weiterbildung 6th, uberarbeitete Aufl.* . Facultas.
Mayring, P. (2016). *Introduction to qualitative social research*. Beltz.
Mayring, P. (2022). *Qualitative Content Analysis: Basics and Techniques* (13th ed.). Beltz.
Moser, C. (2010). *The migration of qualified carers from the new EU member states - a literature analysis and qualitative interviews with Viennese care service managers* [Diploma thesis]. University of Vienna.
Pleschberger, S., & Holzweber, L. (2019). Evaluation of the GuKG amendment 2016. progress report.
Rappold, E., & Juraszovich, B. (2019). Nursing staff demand forecast for Austria.
Rohleder, C. (2012). Demography and demographic change. *Lebenslage und Lebensbewaltigung*, 217.
Rottenhofer, I., Bronneberg, G., Glatz, W., & Steier, A. (2003). *Open curriculum general health care and nursing*. (3851590686). Austrian Federal Institute of Public Health
Schonherr, D. (2021). Working Conditions in Nursing Professions; Special

Evaluation of the Austrian Work Climate Index. *Vienna: Federal Ministry of Social Affairs, Health, Care and Consumer Protection*.

Shaffer, F. A., Bakhshi, M., Cook, K., & Alvarez, T. D. (2022). International nurse recruitment beyond the COVID-19 pandemic: Considerations for the nursing workforce leader. *Nurse Leader*, *20*(2), 161-167.

Ministry of Social Affairs. (2024a). *The health professions register*. Federal Ministry of Social Affairs, Health, Care and Consumer Protection. Retrieved 20.04.2024 from https://www.sozialministerium.at/Themen/Gesundheit/Medizin-und- Gesundheitsberufe/Gesundheitsberuferegister.html

Ministry of Social Affairs. (2024b). *Nostrification of foreign school certificates*.

Federal Ministry of Social Affairs, Health, Care and Consumer Protection. Retrieved 20.04.2024 from

https://www.bmbwf.gv.at/Themen/schule/schulrecht/anauschubi/nostr.html

Stolle-Wahl, C., & Reinhardt, D. (2022). Together against discrimination. *Pflegezeitschrift*, *75*(8), 38-41.

Tahic, Z. (2023). Employment of foreign carers - opportunities and risks for Austria / submitted by Zerina Tahic.

Winter, K., & Sassenberg, K. (2022). Social categorisation, stereotypes, prejudices. *Handbook of peace psychology*.

Witzel, A. (1985). *The problem-centred interview*. Beltz.

Zegelin, A. (2023). Why foreign carers take so long to arrive here. *Pflege Professionell - Das Fachmagazin, 31*.

10 Acknowledgements

I would like to take this opportunity to thank all the people who made my studies and the writing of this thesis possible.

I would especially like to thank Mr Simon Krutter Ph.D., BA for his excellent supervision during the research work. With patience he always answered my questions and shared his expertise and experience with me. As a result, I was able to understand and implement the process of qualitative research.

I would also like to thank my employer for the support and time resources that were made available to me for my studies. Furthermore, for the opportunity to have carried out my research work in the group of companies.

I would like to express my sincere thanks to the interview participants in my study, because without their experience and time, which they made available to me, it would not have been possible to produce this work.

I would like to thank Bernhard, my son's friend, who, as an English teacher, took care of the correct translation of my abstract into English. I would also like to thank my friend Herwig Hutegger for proofreading the entire thesis, who invested many hours in checking my work for grammar and spelling.

I am particularly grateful to my family, as they almost had to do without me for months. Thank you so much for your support with childcare, cooking, shopping, comforting me and keeping me going.

Many thanks also to my dear friend and colleague Bettina, who always managed to cheer me up in difficult times and make me laugh with her special sense of humour.

11 Appendix

Seeboden, 11.12.2023

Information letter and declaration of consent for participation in the study

Dear nursing staff at ,

I am delighted that you are interested in the topic of my work. I am a nursing service manager at and am currently studying on the Health Sciences & Leadership programme at Paracelsus Medical University Salzburg. As part of my studies, I am currently writing my Master's thesis on the topic of **"The integration of new nursing staff from abroad into the nursing service and the team".** The purpose of this letter is to inform you about the aim of the thesis and the procedure. Please read the text carefully. If you have any questions, I will be happy to answer them.

Participation in the study is voluntary and you can withdraw at any time without giving reasons. Refusal to participate or early withdrawal from the study will have no adverse professional or personal consequences for you.

1. Information about the study

The general conditions in the care sector and the prevailing staff shortage require extensive measures to recruit new employees. One solution is the recruitment of nursing staff from abroad, as has been practised in our group for several months. With the integration of colleagues from abroad, there are a number of challenges that need to be overcome, but also opportunities that we should utilise.

What is the purpose of this study?

The aim is to incorporate the concerns, needs and suggestions of existing nursing staff into the integration process and thus improve it and the quality of teamwork.

Why are you being asked to participate?

In order to improve the practical implementation of the integration process in everyday life and to be able to offer you more support in practice, I am looking for experienced care professionals. I would like to ask you to provide me with your knowledge and experience in the form of an expert interview for the preparation of my master's thesis.

to make them available. Expert interviews are a specific form of interview that are interested in very specific bodies of knowledge. In this case, it is about the experience of familiarising migrant nurses from abroad.

Who can take part in the study?

If you meet the criteria below and are interested in participating in the study, I would like to ask you to contact me to participate in the study:

- Qualified carers and care assistants with and without a migration background
- an operating history of at least 1 year
- 5 years of professional experience in Austria

What does participation in the study look like?

I have sent you this letter inviting you to participate in the study on a voluntary basis. Expert interviews lasting approx. 40 minutes are planned with you on site at the care facility or via video conference on your experiences with the induction

and integration of foreign nursing staff.
If you are interested and willing to participate, please contact me and we will agree on the exact time and place.
Before the interview begins, you will first be informed again about the study and everything you can expect in connection with the interview. You will sign a separate consent form. All interviews will be audio-recorded using a digital recording device without mentioning your name or any further indication of your identity. The interviews will be transcribed verbatim and analysed. Instead of your name, a so-called pseudonym will be used and all references to your person will be removed. This makes it impossible for anyone to draw conclusions about you as a person from the written interview. This measure is necessary in order to revoke your participation and to be able to fulfil the requested deletion of your data.

Are there any risks?

There are no risks associated with participation in the study.

Do you have to participate until the end?

You can revoke your willingness to participate and withdraw from the study at any time without giving reasons.

Do you incur any costs or other disadvantages?

There are no costs for you. Apart from the time required to participate, the study has no consequences or disadvantages for you.

2. Data protection

If you have any concerns, questions or complaints about data processing and compliance with data protection requirements, you can of course contact me at any time.
I will take all reasonable steps to ensure the protection of your data in accordance with the General Data Protection Regulation (GDPR) and other laws.

3. What happens to the collected data?

The audio files are deleted after transcription (=transcription into a written form). The pseudonymised data is stored for a period of 10 years.

4. Permission to conduct the study

Permission to conduct the study and the expert interviews was granted by the company management, the head of the Human Resources department and the works council.

5. Declarations of consent

You will receive two declarations of consent with this letter. Please read these at your leisure. I will provide you with more detailed information on the purpose of the survey. If you would like to support my study, please sign both consent forms before you take part in the interview.
I would be very pleased about your voluntary participation! Thank you very much for your support!
With kind regards
Alexandra Konig

Interview guide

Title of the work

The integration of new nursing staff from abroad into the nursing service and the team

Preliminary information

They have been informed about the procedure, the purpose of this interview and the processing of their data. I would also like to inform them that the answers to the questions relate exclusively to their experience of working in the Group. Previous experience on the subject is not part of the study.

1. **How do you see the integration of foreign nursing staff into the nursing service as a solution to the staff shortage in long-term care and what do you understand by the term integration in relation to the nursing service?**

2. **When you think about the induction of new employees, which points are particularly important to you?**

2.1.What should a new carer know about caring for residents and how do you experience day-to-day care when you work in a team with staff from abroad?

2.2.What does nursing documentation mean for them in their everyday work and what benefits do they see in it? What challenges do you face when teaching the key aspects of nursing documentation as a source of information and quality assurance to new foreign nursing professionals?

2.3.When you think about the structures and organisation at your workplace, what does a new employee absolutely need to know? In your opinion, are there any special features when it comes to foreign nursing staff?

2.4.Which people in the company and cooperation partners should a new carer definitely know and why? How does the introduction to these people work in practice?

2.5.When you think of crises and emergency situations, how are the behaviour and procedures in such cases trained in the run-up to induction? How do you experience working with new foreign colleagues in emergencies?

2.6.What is it like for you when you train a new colleague? Does it make a difference to you if they are a foreign carer?

2.7.What time frame did you define for the induction of a new employee? Would you assess the time frame differently for a colleague from abroad and why?

3. In addition to professional training, new specialists should also be integrated into the company, the community and the team. What experiences have you had in this regard and what are the biggest challenges here? What advantages have arisen as a result?

3.1.The nursing profession is one that requires a great deal of communication. How do you see the aspect of "language and profession" in relation to foreign employees? What are the advantages of multilingualism in the team?

3.2.How do they fare when they work with colleagues of foreign origin in the day service?

3.3.When you think of foreign cultures, where do you see challenges in everyday care work? How do you deal with cultural differences when working with new foreign carers? How do you experience the reaction of residents to new carers from other cultures?

3.4.How do they view the personal burden on foreign nursing staff who start work in a foreign country? How do they experience situations in which their foreign colleagues tell them about these burdens?

3.5.What personal impact does the integration of foreign carers have on them? Are there any concerns, fears or worries on their part when several carers of foreign origin are integrated into the team?

4. How do you experience the role of company management or the management of the organisation in the integration of foreign nursing staff?

4.1.In which areas should management provide support for integration?

4.2.What kind of support did you find particularly helpful in the familiarisation and integration of foreign colleagues?

4.3.What information did they receive before new colleagues of foreign origin started work? What information did they want in order to start the integration process well prepared?

4.4.Are there specific measures that you would like to see from the company management, the care service management or the home management?

5. Is there anything else that is important to them with regard to the familiarisation and integration of foreign colleagues? What would you like to see in the future?

interview_4.m4a

I: Well, afterwards I'll say we've discussed everything so far. And I will then start with the first question. How do you see the integration of foreign nursing staff into the nursing service as a solution to the staff shortage?
#00:00:17-2#

B: (...) May I answer? #00:00:24-2#

I: Yes, please. #00:00:24-2#

B: Yes, I actually think it's a really good solution. Above all, it's helped us a lot. We've got two of them and I think it's a really good solution, I have to say. Above all, they both work one hundred per cent, they step in a lot. So it's really, really helped a lot for us. #00:00:54-3#

I: Where are these carers you're talking about? #00:00:59-4#

B: From what kind of country? #00:01:06-4#

I: Yes, exactly. #00:01:06-5#

B: From Tunisia. #00:01:06-5#

I: Do you have others on the team, other carers from other states or other countries? #00:01:15-5#

B: We also have a graduate from Hungary. But otherwise not really, no. #00:01:20-2#

I: What do you generally understand by the term integration in relation to care? #00:01:30-6#

B: Yes, that we don't just have them there to work, but that we really involve them in the team. Like at the Christmas party, that they are there. That they're really involved in the team and are seen as part of it. And yes, also in care, that they are also seen as a member of the care team for the residents and are not seen in any other way. But really quite normally as a carer. So from the residents' point of view and the relatives too, of course. #00:02:17-8#

I: When you think about the induction of new employees, what other points are generally particularly important for them? #00:02:26-9#

B: Firstly, the language is very important. In other words, that you really do have some knowledge of German right from the start. And that the induction programme is held in German as much as possible. Because then you have to be able to speak German with the residents and everything / At some point they have to be able to speak German, for our residents and for their relatives. And that's a big, big point. And I would also give them a bit more familiarisation time so that they really get to know all the residents, all the steps, the procedures. That's simply different here than in other countries. And yes, you simply invest a lot of time, because the better it works then. #00:03:30-5#

Seg. no.	Document name	Code	Segment	Paraphrase	Generalisation
1	B1	Assumption of responsibility	And I also told the [person] that it helps / kindness alone is not enough. I can't do it when he says to me: "It hurts me back there", "Yes, yes, yes, yes." That doesn't work. And if everything is just like that, then it's a problem. As long as there's still a German speaker there, he'll be stuck with it, right? You know, they'll come and I'll speak to them or I'll speak to them once. And then they actually have an easier job, right? They're not burdened with anything. They do their job and are friendly. But that's not enough in geriatric care, is it?	Kindness is not enough. When residents express pain, it's not enough to simply say yes, that doesn't work. If this is the general approach, it's a problem. Existing carers are burdened with the responsibility for this. Foreign carers do the planned work and are friendly. Too few in geriatric care	Health complaints of the residents: • No reaction in the event of pain, only "Yes" is answered. • If no one from the existing care team is available, there is no intervention in the event of residents' health complaints. Relying on existing carers: • Exposure of existing carers to all residents' health complaints. • If time is of the essence, nursing males are passed on to existing carers. Resident needs: • No attentiveness to residents' needs, e.g. whether sufficient food was served • Neglecting basic care activities such as personal hygiene when under time pressure. Care documentation: • Nursing malpractice is not documented, which means that the
2	B2	Assumption of	So, I see more of an	I see a lack of responsibility	

		responsibility	egalitarianism, gg? People actually rely more on whoever is there, gg? Because they don't feel as responsible. They do what they can, gg? And the other, well, the second one is there, gg? And what doesn't work, doesn't work. So if it doesn't work out over time, then it works itself out	in relying on the existing nursing staff. No sense of responsibility, they do what they can. They leave everything else to existing carers. Activities that don't run out of time are neglected.	

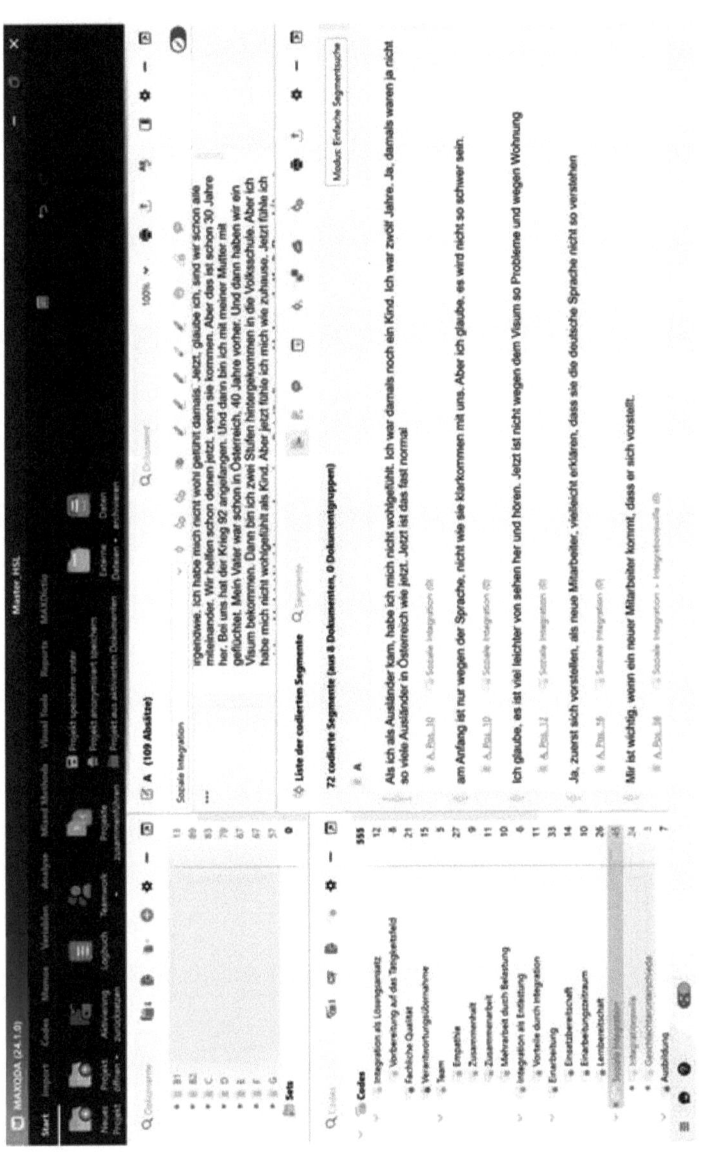
MAXQDA (24.1.0)
Master_HSL
A (109 Absätze)
Soziale Integration
irgendwie. Ich habe mich nicht wohl gefühlt damals. Jetzt, glaube ich, sind wir schon alle miteinander. Wir helfen schon denen jetzt, wenn sie kommen. Aber das ist schon 30 Jahre her. Bei uns hat der Krieg 92 angefangen. Und dann bin ich mit meiner Mutter mit geflüchtet. Mein Vater war schon in Österreich, 40 Jahre vorher. Und dann haben wir ein Visum bekommen. Dann bin ich zwei Stufen hintergekommen in die Volksschule. Aber ich habe mich nicht wohlgefühlt als Kind. Aber jetzt fühle ich mich wie zuhause. Jetzt fühle ich
Liste der codierten Segmente
72 codierte Segmente (aus 8 Dokumenten, 0 Dokumentgruppen)
Modus: Einfache Segmentsuche
Als ich als Ausländer kam, habe ich mich nicht wohlgefühlt. Ich war damals noch ein Kind. Ich war zwölf Jahre. Ja, damals waren ja nicht so viele Ausländer in Österreich wie jetzt. Jetzt ist das fast normal
am Anfang ist nur wegen der Sprache, nicht wie sie klarkommen mit uns. Aber ich glaube, es wird nicht so schwer sein.
Ich glaube, es ist viel leichter von sehen her und hören. Jetzt ist nicht wegen dem Visum so Probleme und wegen Wohnung
Ja, zuerst sich vorstellen, als neue Mitarbeiter, vielleicht erklären, dass sie die deutsche Sprache nicht so verstehen
Mir ist wichtig, wenn ein neuer Mitarbeiter kommt, dass er sich vorstellt.
Codes 555
Integration als Lösungsansatz 12
Vorbereitung auf das Tätigkeitsfeld 8
Fachliche Qualität 21
Verantwortungsübernahme 15
Team 5
Empathie 27
Zusammenhalt 9
Zusammenarbeit 11
Mehrarbeit durch Belastung 10
Integration als Entlastung 6
Vorteile durch Integration 11
Einarbeitung 33
Einsatzbereitschaft 14
Einarbeitungszeitraum 10
Lernbereitschaft 26
Ausbildung 7

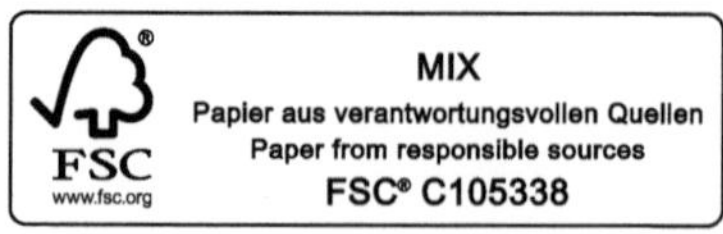

Printed by Books on Demand GmbH, Norderstedt / Germany